The
Lazy Girl's
Guide to Good
Health

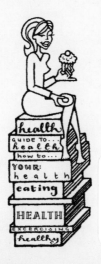

D1362318

Anita Naik is a freelance journalist who has written for *New Woman*, *M Magazine*, *Cosmopolitan*, *Glamour*, *Now* and *Men's Health*. She specialises in health, sex and relationships and is currently the sex columnist for *More* magazine.

The Lazy Girl's Guide to Good Health

Anita Naik

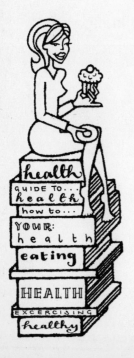

PIATKUS

✿ Visit the Piatkus website!

Piatkus publishes a wide range of bestselling fiction and non-fiction, including books on health, mind, body & spirit, sex, self-help, cookery, biography and the paranormal.

If you want to:
- read descriptions of our popular titles
- buy our books over the internet
- take advantage of our special offers
- enter our monthly competition
- learn more about your favourite Piatkus authors

VISIT OUR WEBSITE AT: **www.piatkus.co.uk**

Copyright © 2002 by Anita Naik

First published in 2002 by
Judy Piatkus (Publishers) Limited
5 Windmill Street
London W1T 2JA

Reprinted 2002 (twice), 2003

The moral right of the author has been asserted

A catalogue record for this book is available from the British Library

ISBN 0 7499 2253 2

Text design by skeisch
Edited by Cathy Herbert
Cover and inside illustrations by Nicola Cramp

This book has been printed on paper manufactured with respect for the environment using wood from managed sustainable resources

Typeset by Palimpsest Book Production, Polmont, Stirlingshire
Printed and bound in Great Britain by Biddles Ltd, *www.biddles.co.uk*

contents

acknowledgements

For all their advice and encouragement, thanks goes to my family, my agent Judy Chilcote, and my two incredibly non-lazy friends – Jenni Baxter and Julie Sleaford. Very special appreciation goes out to the many lazy girls who inspired this book, most especially, Jane 'I'm idle' Coleman, Laurie 'But I've no time to do that' Zulauf and Alison 'I need my sleep' Ive. Note to them (and all other lazy girls I know and love) – please read this book, learn it by heart, and stop asking me why you can't get into your jeans.

introduction

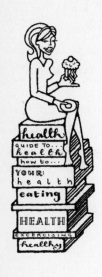

Why this book can help you

'Is it just me,' one of my friends asked recently, 'or have hangovers become more painful?' If you know what we're talking about, it's likely you also live a life of 21st-century debauchery. A life where sleep is something you catch up on at weekends, exercise something you once did at school, and healthy eating a fad you attempt every time your knickers get too tight.

If so, good health is probably the last thing on your mind, or something you imagine you'll get round to one day when age sets in and there's nothing to watch on TV. Who can blame you? Life probably seems far too short to forgo chocolate in favour of multivitamins, drink herbal tea instead of cappuccinos, and give up nights out for 40 minutes on the treadmill.

Well, this isn't the bit where I say – 'Aha! But that's how you have to live if you want to get to your 65th birthday without a Zimmer frame.' This is where I point out that being healthy, though relatively time-consuming and irritating, isn't difficult. Even the laziest girl can re-haul her wellbeing without radically changing her life. Roughly translated this doesn't necessarily mean a 28-day detox of brown rice and water, a strict regime of food elimination, enlisting the help of a personal trainer (although I have to admit these are essential if you're a spectacularly lazy being), or starvation tactics. All it takes are a few simple changes, preferably involving both action and thought – changes that will help you get over those killer hangovers, deal with your skin breakouts, beat fatigue, sort out your sex problems, and zap those anxieties about whether or not to have dessert.

This is where *A Lazy Girl's Guide* comes in. Unlike other health books, you won't find any pseudo-scientific nonsense in here. I won't be advocating a personality bypass or telling you to get to bed by 10 pm. I wouldn't dare to suggest you give up everything you like just so you can have the body of a goddess. This book is about manageable health. It may not transform you into a Brazilian supermodel but it will make you feel 100% better, give you more energy and help you to live the way you want. I've taken a back-to-basics approach, which works on the premise that we all overlook the obvious because we assume we know it already. This isn't to say you won't learn anything new – because I've included plenty of advanced tips for those of you who already have a pile of health books propping up a table somewhere.

Finally, you can take this book in a number of ways. You can read it on a dip in/dip out basis – focusing on what's bothering you – or you can read it from front to back. While the cover-to-cover approach is best because – let's face it – health is about the whole picture, you can use this book any way you want.

If you're still asking yourself, 'Why should I bother?', ponder this: good health equals a stronger sex drive, more stamina, less wrinkles, better moods and, best of all, masses of energy – essential if, like the rest of us, you're planning to grow old loudly, disgracefully, and for as long as possible.

chapter 1
The body stuff

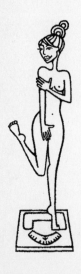

How healthy is healthy? Most of us ask ourselves this question at some point. Healthy enough to squeeze into a size 10 pair of jeans? Healthy enough to run for a bus, without passing out? Or healthy enough to wear a vest top without worrying about breast and tummy spillage? How about fat? Is being fat being able to pinch more than an inch (if so 98% of the UK population are in trouble), being unable to climb the stairs, or having to buy a calorie counters sandwich for lunch every day?

Statistics show that as a nation we are turning into a sack of lumpy couch potatoes and getting fatter and fatter, simply because we're eating too much and not taking enough exercise. Bizarrely enough, we're also devouring health foods and calorie counting meals by the bucket load, and joining gyms all over the place. So why is it that we just can't get our heads around weight issues, healthy eating and exercise?

Well, it's probably because healthy living sounds far too much like hard work. The story goes – cut out everything you like to eat, drink and do, and take up everything you loathe. Ditch the pizza for a lettuce salad, wash it down with some tasty water, do three aerobics classes a week and never get drunk. Is it worth it? Most of us think not.

But taking up healthy eating and regular exercise doesn't have to mean morphing into a health fanatic or getting smug about your lifestyle. Unsure of the state of your health? Start by asking yourself the following:

Do You Often:

- Sleep through your alarm clock
- Feel irritable mid-morning
- Tired after lunch
- Fatigued by 3 pm
- Bloated after most meals
- Sluggish by 8 pm
- Lacking in energy all day

Is It Getting Harder To:

- Get over a hangover
- Get over a late night
- Drink mid-afternoon and get away with it
- Find the energy to go out at night

- Get off the sofa once you're watching TV
- Eat a takeaway without triggering some kind of digestion problem
- Get into your old clothes
- Live the way you want to and still get into work on time

If you've answered yes to any (or all) of the above, it's worth considering that fatigue, lack of energy, bad digestion and an inability to dance the night away without sleeping for days afterwards, are not problems that occur naturally with age.

However, they will if you don't think about how you're fuelling your body. If you put low-grade petrol into a Grand Prix Ferrari, it won't be of Grand Prix calibre for long. Roughly translated this means: feed your body with booze, takeaways, packets of crisps and cups of coffee and your body will retaliate.

How healthy living will affect your health

Give you more energy

Take it from me, when your system is working at its full potential, you're likely to wake up before your alarm rings, feel refreshed when you do get up and stay relatively

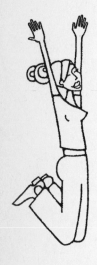

fatigue-free until bedtime. On top of this, you'll be clear-headed and have no need for large cups of black coffee. Sadly, 80% of the population don't feel this way because they chow down on comforting stodge and processed foods, heavy in fat and hidden sugars. Heavily refined foods (processed meals and junk food) turn to sugar more quickly in the body, leading to very high and very low blood sugar levels. This in turn gives you energy highs and lows, which eventually lead to horrible mid-afternoon slumps.

Lazy fix one: Avoid a chocolate fix. If you crave sweet stuff, stick to fruit (high in natural sugar), honey on toast (natural sugar and carbohydrate – good for energy) and, if you have to, good quality dark chocolate.

Lazy fix two: Reduce your coffee and alcohol intake. Boring, I know, but the energy surge these stimulants give you is followed by an energy low. Worse still, they're addictive – meaning you need to drink more and more to get the same effect. Drink more water instead. A couple of glasses in between your cappuccinos will dilute the effect.

Lazy fix three: Eat little and often, i.e. once every three hours. This will keep your blood sugar level up, keeping your energy on an even keel.

Give you fab digestion

Does irritable bowel syndrome plague your life? (For more on this, see Chapter 5.) Do you feel bloated, constipated, full of wind, or suffer from diarrhoea and/or indigestion? Are you constantly complaining about tiredness and stomach aches? If so, 'you are what you eat'. For your digestion to work properly you need to start off with the right types of food.

Lazy fix one: Avoid foods that make you go. Certain foods, fruits and drinks, like coffee, tea, alcohol and sugar-laden foods have an unhealthy laxative, so steer clear of them.

Lazy fix two: Cut down on the junk. Processed, fatty and sugary foods should all be enjoyed with caution as they can slow down your digestion.

Lazy fix three: Add variety to your diet. Eating the same foods every day is the kiss of death to your stomach and probably why it's playing up. Eat a little bit of everything and bear in mind that while fibre is essential, too much will cause wind, bloating and pain.

Keep you flu-free

Your immune system exists to stop bacteria and viruses from invading your body and making you ill. If you find you're susceptible to every cold and flu bug going around or that you always have a sniffle or sore throat, it's worth remembering that your immune system relies directly on the food you give it to function properly. When you skip meals, eat food that has no nutritious value and swap meals for booze, you're asking for a shut down. As well as successive colds, a slow immune system can also lead to fatigue and food intolerances.

Lazy fix one: Drink more fluids. Boost your immunity by drinking more water as this will help to flush out germs, bacteria and even colds.

Lazy fix two: Choose fish dishes. Eat more oily fish, such as salmon, tuna and mackerel. It's rich in Omega 3 and 6, the fatty acids essential for good immunity.

Lazy fix three: Eat an orange a day. Oranges are rich in both vitamin C and antioxidants and will give you an immunity boost.

Keep you happy

Believe it or not, certain foods make you grumpy. Too much sugar, for instance, can give you a high followed by a low. Too much coffee can lead to anxiety and irritability (see Chapter 3), and not enough protein can lead to fatigue.

Lazy fix one: Eat something raw. Reduce the amount of refined and processed foods you eat and replace them with fresh and raw foods – it's cheap, it's easy and you don't have to cook them!

tips

Eat a piece of fruit a day. It is rich in anti-oxidants and will help you stay young and healthy.

Lazy fix two: Think about your bread intake. Many women suffer from wheat intolerance, which leads to low mood, stomach problems and fatigue – this is usually because they eat wheat at every single meal: cereal for breakfast, a sandwich for lunch and pasta for dinner. If this sounds like your average day, cut back or even cut out the bread, pasta and cereal for a while.

Lazy fix three: Give yourself a break from sugar (instead of a sugar break). Don't succumb to sugar cravings more than once a day or your blood sugar levels will keep rising and falling, and you'll find yourself dozing at your desk.

Give you regular periods

Your cycle length, PMS and periods are all affected by what you weigh, and what you eat. To discover your healthy weight, forget about standing on your bathroom scales and work out what's known as your Body Mass Index (BMI), the scale now used by all health professionals. This works by assessing your weight in relation to your height and tells you how healthy your current shape is.

Work out your Body Mass Index

Divide your weight in kilograms by your height in metres squared (1 lb = 0.45 kg and there are 14 lb in a stone. 1 ft = 30.48 cm).

So if you weigh 10 stones and are 5 ft 6:

First work out what you weigh in kilograms:	140 lb x 0.45 kg= 63 kg
Then work out your height in metres:	5.6 x 30.48 cm = 1.7 m
Square your height:	1.70 x 1.70 = 2.89
Then divide your weight, 63 kg, by your height squared, 2.89	= a BMI of 21

A BMI of 20 is considered underweight and is likely to mean sporadic periods or no periods at all. This is because oestrogen, the hormone that causes ovulation, needs body fat in order to be produced.

A BMI of over 25 is considered overweight and will make your periods irregular and heavy, because your body is producing too much oestrogen.

Lazy fix one: Get your weight right for you. Losing just a small amount of weight (we're not talking major diet here), or gaining a bit could make all the difference to your periods and PMS. You don't have to stick to a chart, just go by what feels comfortable for you.

Lazy fix two: Avoid caffeine, alcohol and sugary foods near your period. Do this five days before your period and during it and you'll reduce period pain, bloating and pre-menstrual headaches.

Lazy fix three: Be sensible about what you do to yourself. Don't over-exercise or crash diet near your period. It will throw your cycle into disarray and make you feel pretty horrible.

The truth about dieting

Admit it, you're probably thinking about a diet right now. Most of us are, even if we're too lazy to do anything about it. In fact, if figures are to be believed, never have so many of us wanted to be quite so thin so fast. Worldwide expenditure per year on diet products is enormous (£2 billion in the UK). The desire to ease the agony of trips to the bathroom scales means even the super-fit people I know will consider any bizarre diet going. So, just in case you're tempted, here's the lowdown on why you've got a fat chance of losing any weight on the so-called 'super' diets.

"never have so many of us wanted to be quite so thin so fast."

DIETS DON'T WORK ON A LONG-TERM BASIS BECAUSE ... starving your body of calories (which is essentially what all diets do) causes your metabolism to slow down and cling onto everything you eat, making it harder for you to lose weight and stay on the diet.

However, you can also ignore that depressing '95% of people who lose weight will put it back on' statistic. A new survey from the *International Journal of Obesity* shows that the reality is actually four times better than this – meaning that if you do shift your unwanted weight, you're likely to keep it off for much longer than you think (if not for ever).

It's also worth pointing out that everyone's weight can fluctuate by as much as 1.5 kg (about 3 lb) a day thanks to the menstrual cycle and associated water retention. So don't torture yourself with daily weigh ins – the only thing they'll do is have you reaching for comfort food or a faddy diet. The lazy way to weigh yourself successfully is to go by the fit of your clothes.

Lazy girl's guide to diets

1. Protein-only diets
This was the first real diet to reach superstardom status. Published way back in 1961, it sold over 20 million, and it's still the hot celeb fave because it promises quick results with little effort (though it's tough to do). The idea is to eat protein-only foods so that something known as 'ketosis' occurs in the body. This is a condition whereby the body begins breaking down everything such as

your lean muscle mass in order to get energy – and so you lose weight.

The problem is that protein-only diets are extremely unhealthy – so much so that over 10,000 doctors and dieticians at a recent US Eating Disorders conference condemned them. Apparently, choosing to chow down on bacon, steaks, burgers, eggs and cheese, over potatoes, bread and pasta is bad for your health (as if you didn't know that!). Unsavoury side effects of this diet include bad breath, mammoth fatigue, heart disease and kidney and liver damage. Plus, can you imagine never being able to eat bread, potatoes, pasta, rice and/or noodles ever again?

2. Fruit-only diets

Fruit is good for you, right? Yes, but not if it's the only thing you eat for two weeks. The fact is that while this diet can cause rapid weight loss because it's so low in calories, it also causes fainting, dizziness, ample amounts of time on the toilet and headaches. Another one condemned by doctors everywhere.

3. Weight loss drugs

Xenical (Orlistat), the new anti-obesity drug available on the NHS, has a huge success rate. However, it's only prescribed to people who are actually obese. It works by preventing fat from being absorbed in the body, but it's no miracle solution. Alongside the drug (taken in pill form), patients have to follow a very strict low calorie diet. Secret snacking can result in anal leakage and diarrhoea.

4. Meal replacements

The bad news about meal replacements is that they never teach you to eat properly, which means the second you go back to your old ways the weight reappears. Plus they are too low in calories, boring to maintain (no real food until 6 pm), and cause headaches, dizziness, lack of energy and bad breath.

5. Extreme detox diets

Detox dieters aim to lose 7 kg (14 lbs) or more in a month by eating squirrel food, vegetables, fruit and water. Well, apart from the fact that this is dull, dull, dull, it's not good for your overall health to lose more than a kilogram (2 lbs) a week. While on this type of diet you may experience headaches, bad skin, bad breath, fatigue and a very bad temper.

6. Liposuction

You could always save up and have your fat cut out – like the 15,000 people who underwent liposuction in the UK last year, and the 400,000 Americans who'll do the same this year. The scary fact is that this procedure was never designed to be a weight cure, but a way of getting rid of sneaky bits of fat that couldn't be zapped with exercise and dieting. Far from being an easy and pain-free solution, liposuction hurts, comes with complications and can kill you. Plus, if you keep on eating badly, the fat will come back on, but in new places around the trimmed bits, giving you a weird bumpy look.

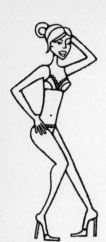

The truth about weight loss

Want to know how to lose weight fast and for good? Well, all you have to do is this – EAT LESS AND DO MORE.

This is basically what all the half-a-million diet books currently on the market are telling you to do. It's a known scientific equation – eat more calories than you expend and you'll gain weight! Consume fewer calories and burn more off and you'll lose weight and keep it off.

The best way to do this is to aim to lose about a kilogram (2 lbs) a week – which is easier than you think. If you're someone who eats too much junk, take the two foods you eat the most – for example, bread and pasta – and replace them for four weeks with something else (except not cake, chips and chocolate because this is supposed to be a weight loss programme). By changing the food you eat, you'll consume less and lose weight.

If you like to eat the same food at every meal and can't get to grips with the replacement idea, try to break your meals up. Eating less but more often makes your metabolism work more efficiently. Break your three meals up into five smaller meals. Not only will this help you eat less, you'll also never be hungry.

Get yourself a healthy body without starving, or exerting yourself that much

Whether you're overweight, underweight or normal weight, if you survive on takeaway pizza, think powdered mash potato is a food group and/or choose booze over food, you don't have a healthy attitude to eating.

You may not want to be a healthy eating goddess but that doesn't mean you have to be Waynetta Slob when it comes to your diet. The trick is simple – forget about reading the healthy eating books, listening to endless expert advice and mulling over nutrition studies in the newspapers – just start eating as much raw, natural and fresh food as possible. Eat when you're hungry and choose food that you really want to eat, not think you should eat. The result – believe it or not – is that you'll get the body you want. For more tips read on . . .

1. Admit to how much you eat

Most of us eat way too much, and that's why we put on weight. It sounds obvious but, when asked, most people claim they hardly eat anything. Be honest – think of every morsel you put in your mouth each day . . . it all adds up.

2. Stop yo-yo dieting

Roller coaster dieting carries potential health hazards, including an increased risk of heart disease and diabetes. In case that doesn't persuade you to stop, it also equals a decreased metabolic rate, a greater taste for fatty foods and a loss of lean muscle mass.

3. Boost your self-esteem

Yes, that old chestnut. If your self-esteem has been eaten away by your body issues, it's time to think about how you can build it up. Eating disorder studies show that people who aren't fixated about having the 'perfect' body or being an ideal weight are happier and have healthier diets.

4. Develop an inner coach

Give your internal weight critic the boot in favour of a more supportive voice. If you find it difficult, try asking yourself this – would you be so unkind to a friend?

5. Everything counts

Don't be someone who thinks, 'What's the point, I'm fat anyway?' Everything counts when it comes to healthy eating and exercise. Climbing stairs, taking the dog for a walk each night for 30 minutes, eating low fat until dinner time, not having that 4 pm chocolate biscuit and opting for a diet mixer in your vodka.

6. Eat chocolate if you want to

Yes, you read that right – chocolate in itself isn't bad for your diet (unless, of course, you're going through a family sized bar every day). It actually triggers the release of your brain's pleasure chemicals, known as endorphins, which will improve your mood and strengthen your immunity. If you're going to eat loads of the stuff, however, it's better to opt for high quality, where the cocoa solids are higher (70%) and the sugar content lower – this will have the added bonus of controlling your blood sugar, meaning no horrible mood swings. Plus, good quality dark chocolate contains beneficial antioxidants that fight off free radicals (molecules that destroy cells in the body), which have been shown to contribute towards ageing and age-related diseases. It's also worth noting that chocolate contains iron (good for tiredness), calcium (good for strong bones and PMS) and magnesium (also good for PMS). PS: It doesn't give you spots (and that's official – just ask your doctor)!

7. Eat breakfast every day

The reason behind this advice is simple – your body needs fuel in the morning. Not only has it not eaten for at least ten hours, research shows that those who skip breakfast lack concentration at work, eat more at lunch, and snack more during the day because they haven't revved up their metabolism. Don't feel hungry in the morning or can't be bothered to pour out a bowl of cereal? The answer is to get into a routine. Prepare what you want for breakfast the night before, set your alarm 15 minutes earlier and at least drink a glass of juice before you walk out the door. Experts say if you make yourself do this for a week, by week two you'll be ready to add a piece of toast or cereal to the mix – and bingo, you're eating breakfast!

8. Eat some protein every day

At least 25% of your daily food intake should be protein because it's essential for building bones, healthy teeth, hair and nails. It's

tips

Research shows that those who skip breakfast end up gaining more weight than those who eat before work.

also vital for healthy blood and maintaining your blood sugar levels. The best sources are chicken, fish, soya products, milk and eggs. A diet rich in protein (as opposed to protein-only) will control your appetite and stimulate the hormone glucagon, which burns fat in the body. Plus, all you mid-afternoon slumpers, a lunch rich in protein rather than carbohydrate (pasta, potato, bread) will keep your energy levels up until dinner.

9. Eat carbohydrates every day

There are two types of carbohydrates – complex carbs and simple carbs. A simple carbohydrate is any grain that has been processed to change it from its original state, e.g. bread or pasta. Eat too much of the simple carbohydrates and you'll feel tired and sluggish because this kind of food is converted into sugar very quickly by the body. To achieve weight loss and feel healthy, nutritionists suggest that our meals should always contain both forms of carbohydrate. One third should be complex – vegetables and grains – and a smaller portion should be simple – potato, rice or pasta.

10. Eat fat every day

Not all dietary fat is bad for you. The body needs unsaturated fat for cell growth, fertility, healthy periods and skin. It's also essential for hormones and healthy bones. This means you can't afford to cut all fat from your diet. If you're still tempted, consider this – unsaturated fat can aid weight loss by turning off your hunger signals. The best unsaturated fats are Omega 3 and 6 fatty acids, found in oily fish, nuts and seeds. Deficiency signs are dry skin, low energy and mood swings. Saturated fats, found in meat, butter and hard margarine, are the bad fats that can cause heart disease and should be eaten with extreme caution.

11. Check your servings

The recommended daily servings are: 6 portions of grain (bread and cereal), 5–7 portions of fruit and vegetables, 2–3 of dairy and 2–3 of protein. This might sound like a huge amount, but a serving is much less than you think.

Guide to servings

- apple = 1 serving
- glass of fruit juice = 1 serving
- 125g (40 oz) of cooked vegetables = 1 serving (so a normal dinner portion of runner beans is already 2 servings)
- 65g (20 oz) of dried fruit = 1 serving
- baked potato = 1 serving
- bagel = 2–3 servings
- 2–3 tbsp of pasta = 1 serving
- matchbox sized piece of cheese = 1 serving
- small pot of yoghurt = 1 serving
- glass of milk = 1 serving
- cheese and salad sandwich with fruit juice and an apple = 2 servings of grain, 3 servings of fruit and vegetables and 2 servings of dairy

12. Snack away

To snack or not to snack, that is the question! Well, the truth is it's impossible not to snack. Plus, it's natural to feel hungry every few hours, so if you're dying for something to eat between meals, the chances are your body's telling you that you need fuel. What to eat is the real question. While it might be tempting to pop down to the newsagent's and grab a bar of something, it's wise to choose your snacks more carefully. You could probably get away with a sugar snack in the morning, but taking one mid-afternoon could be lethal to your energy levels. For healthier mid-afternoon food, think fruit, cheese and nuts.

13. Watch your portions

If, like most of us, you can't be bothered to weigh your food, the chances are you're eating too much at one sitting. You can eat as many vegetables (except for potatoes) as you want, but be careful with fruit. Some fruit is very high in sugar – avoid too much pineapple, banana, mango and passion fruit if you want to lose weight. Instead, stick to hard fruits and perennials like apples and pears. As for portions of meat and fish – it's simple – never eat any piece of protein that's bigger than the palm of your hand.

14. Don't ban foods

The fastest way to eat unhealthily is to divide your foods into good and bad ones. Apart from encouraging obsessive behaviour around eating, it invites a binge mentality. Ban all chocolate and all you'll think about is chocolate, chocolate and chocolate. Allow

tips

Avoid lots of sugar-loaded fruits if you want to lose weight.

yourself a small bar once a day and you'll be satiated. The truth is that there are no good or bad foods.

15. Drink more water

Research shows that three out of four people are dehydrated. The average adult needs eight glasses a day (2 litres) because we lose 3.5 litres (about 6 pints) a day through urinating, breathing and sweating. You probably think you can't drink this amount. Actually, it's only half a glass every hour that you're awake, or two gulps every half an hour.

16. Take some vitamins and minerals

In an ideal world we'd get all our nutrients from our diet and wouldn't need extra help. Sadly, these days lots of foods have been robbed of their nutrients in the preparation process, so it helps to help yourself. For those who can't be bothered to work it out, a multivitamin covers all bases. For specific vitamins and minerals, and their uses, see below:

vitamins and minerals

Vitamin/ Mineral	What you need them for	Recommended daily amount (RDA)
B vitamins	hormone production, easier periods and your brain	1.2 mg
vitamin C	healthy immune system	50 mg

Vitamin/ Mineral	What you need them for	Recommended daily amount (RDA)
vitamin D	healthy bones and hair	10 mg
vitamin E	healthy skin	3 mg
iron	energy and healthy periods	15 mg
calcium	healthy bones and teeth	700 mg
zinc	good for your immune system and essential for healthy fertility	30 mg

17. Don't skip meals

Do you crave sugary foods halfway through the day? Feel like you could sleep at your desk after lunch? Feel irritable if you can't eat as soon as you're hungry? If so, what you eat could be to blame. When you eat too much starch or sugar, the body's blood sugar level rises too fast and the body responds to calm it down. This then causes blood sugar levels to fall, causing instant fatigue and crankiness. The trick is to eat smaller meals, more often, and to not skip meals.

"eat smaller meals, more often, and don't skip meals."

18. Cut down on salt

Cutting your salt levels can help you maintain a healthy diet in more ways than you think. Most importantly, it will lower your blood pressure and lessen your chances of heart disease. The way to do it is simple – eat less processed foods (they all contain high levels of salt), drink less fizzy diet drinks, and don't add salt to your food. Though it will taste weird at first, within a few days you won't notice it and if you cut out processed snacks, you'll feel less fatigued and be more likely to lose weight.

Eat junk successfully

Okay, so you don't want to give up your nights out, takeaways and restaurant meals. Here's how to eat fast food without ending up as fat as a Christmas turkey:

Indian Food

Avoid: pickles – they are steeped in oil; poppadums – they are deep fried; creamy curries – they are steeped in cream and coconut, which are both high in fat; pilau rice – it is cooked in ghee (clarified butter).
Opt for: tandoori or tikka chicken/fish dishes, as these are oven baked and low in fat; plain rice.

The Late Night Kebab

Avoid: the doner – it's greasy and fatty; the extra bag of chips; the fizzy cola.
Opt for: the chicken kebab – it's grilled and low in fat; salad with no dressing.

Pizza

Avoid: thin crust, twisted crust, cheese crust – they are all heaped with extra fat.

Opt for: thick crust (or thin if baked in a wood oven); ask for less cheese and swap in alternative toppings like vegetables, egg, fish or chicken.

Chinese Food

Avoid: egg fried rice, spring rolls, fried noodles and crispy duck – they are all steeped in fat.

Opt for: plain rice, boiled vermicelli rice noodles, stir fried chicken, fish dishes and vegetables.

Chocolate

Avoid: creamy fillings and extra fillings – it's just extra sugar and fat; family sized bars (yes, you will eat it all); bars with biscuits inside – again, it's extra fat.

Opt for: a bar of plain or milk chocolate – it will give you the taste you want without the extra sugar.

Ice Cream

Avoid: American style weird-named ice creams stuffed with bits of chocolate, biscuits, fudge and marshmallows.

Opt for: American style frozen yoghurt – it tastes the same and has half the fat and sugar.

Italian

Avoid: creamy pasta sauces; added cheese; olives; garlic bread.

Opt for: vegetable sauces, chicken or fish grills with salads; ciabatta bread.

American Fast Food

Avoid: the double and triple whammies with cheese, mayo and extra fries with a milkshake.

Opt for: a smaller sized hamburger without mayo and cheese, but have two and delete the extra fries.

"only 1% of people can blame their weight on their parents."

Good Old English Fry Ups

Avoid: fried bacon, fried sausages, fried eggs, fried bread.

Opt for: grilled bacon, grilled sausages, scrambled eggs, toast, grilled mushrooms.

Café Breakfast

Avoid: full-fat lattes and muffins.

Opt for: skimmed milk, cappuccinos and skinny bran muffins

Weight loss myths

Myth: *You have to have your main meal at lunch time*

While it's true that sloth-like couch potatoes need to eat their main meal at lunch so that the body has a chance to burn at least some food off before sleeping, people who do even a little bit of exercise can eat meals at any time of day because the body's muscles will carry on burning food as fuel all day long.

Myth: *Calories from fat make you fatter than calories from carbohydrates*
Eat more carbohydrates than you can burn off and you'll end up gaining weight because, at the end of the day, calories are calories, wherever they come from.

Myth: *People who are overweight have slower metabolisms*
Overweight people have faster metabolisms because they need to burn off more energy to keep going. However, they don't get thin because they eat too much and don't do enough exercise.

Myth: *Size is hereditary*
Only 1% of the population can blame their parents. Currently 40% of the UK population is overweight.

Myth: *You can eat as much as you want as long as it's fat-free or low fat*
Fat-free doesn't mean calorie-free or sugar-free, and low fat doesn't mean low calorie, so both can make you gain weight.

Myth: *You can diet without doing any exercise*
You can, but you'll lose weight quicker if you boost your metabolic rate through exercise.

Myth: *A vegetarian diet is less fattening*
It's not necessarily healthier or less fattening – many vegetarians eat too much fat, such as cheese. In any case, meat (even red meat) is low fat if you eat a lean cut.

Myth: *Eating late makes you put on weight*
Not true – it's your calorie intake for the day that counts, not when you eat. Eating at midnight won't make you any fatter than eating at 8 pm.

Myth: *Eating breakfast makes you hungrier*
Eating breakfast kick starts your metabolism, and though you are hungry by lunch, this is good news because it means you have been burning calories all morning and need food for energy, not because it's lunch time.

Is your healthy eating out of hand?

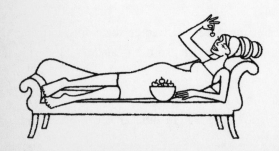

Having spent the whole chapter so far talking about healthy eating, I should point out that even the laziest girl can make healthy eating an unhealthy obsession and thereby lose all the benefits of eating well.

Are you too healthy?

- Since you started eating healthily have you suffered from any of the following: headaches, bad skin, light headedness or period problems?
- Do you find that you keep getting stricter with your diet?
- Do you take pride in telling people what you do and don't eat?
- Do your friends complain that you are too awkward to cook for?
- Do you grill the waitress about menu options in a restaurant and then ask for something not on the menu?
- Do you purposely stay at home to avoid unhealthy eating options at friends' houses?

If you have answered yes to more than two of the above, you are turning into a food Nazi. Three or more, you should think about giving yourself some food freedom. Yes to all of the above – you need to seek advice from a therapist specialising in food disorders.

How healthy eating can damage your health

Being too preoccupied with healthy eating and cutting out food groups is a sign that your diet isn't healthy.

Cut out fat and . . . your periods will stop because fat levels will decrease in the body and oestrogen production will be cut back. Unsaturated fat (found in oily fish and olive oil) is an essential part of good health. It aids digestion, boosts immunity and, in the right proportions, helps keep your heart healthy.

Cut out carbohydrate and . . . your energy levels will deplete. Eventually your body will start taking nourishment from your lean muscle mass in an attempt to enable you to do everyday things like run up the stairs.

Cut out dairy and . . . you will starve your body of adequate calcium and open the doors to osteoporosis – the brittle bone disease that affects one in three post-menopausal women. Bone mass peaks at the age of 35. After this point, 1% of bone mass is lost every year, more if adequate supplies of calcium are not routed to support the bones in the body.

Cut out protein and . . . your skin, nails, bones and hair will start to fall apart. You'll lack energy and feel massively tired.

25 ways to boost your diet

1 Read Food Labels
Don't be fooled – 80% fat-free means it's still 20% full of fat, which is pretty high. 'No added sugar' doesn't mean sugar-free, and 'low fat' doesn't mean low calorie. Read your labels carefully for exact measures and a better indication of what you're eating.

2 Add Seeds To Your Diet
Linseed, flax seeds, pumpkin and sunflower seeds are all rich in Omega 3 and 6 and can help stabilise your hormone levels, giving you less painful periods and reducing your risk of heart disease.

3 Eat More Cereal
A recent study showed you could lose up to 2 kg (4 lbs) in two weeks if you eat something like cornflakes for breakfast and lunch and then add a daily snack and a normal dinner to the mix. A little dull but it could help get you on a healthier track.

4 Eat Apples
It will improve your digestion and your fitness levels by boosting your lung capacity, thanks to the antioxidant quercetin found within its flesh.

5 Beat Bloated And Windy Days
Think about what you eat. Fizzy drinks, carbonated water, beans, lentils, cabbage, broccoli and fruit right after a meal can ferment in your stomach and cause painful digestion. However, a certain amount of wind is normal – help yourself by eating more slowly (less swallowed air) and eating bio yoghurt to aid digestion.

6 Take Your Vitamins With Your Meals
Not instead of a meal, or you're wasting your money. Remember, vitamins are there to up your nutrient intake not replace food. It's also worth noting that many vitamins and minerals are better absorbed if taken with food that has some fat content.

7 Eat Cancer Protecting Foods

Leafy green vegetables, like cabbage and sprouts, and soya contain chemicals that actively protect you from cancer. In soya foods there is something known as an isoflavone that slows down the growth of cancer cells.

8 Boost Digestion

If you suffer from a slow digestive system that makes you feel lethargic, tired and gripey – it's likely you need to drink more. The bowel needs plenty of fluid in order to detoxify. Help yourself by having at least two glasses of water between meals.

9 Think About What You Are Drinking

We all know alcohol adds calories and fat, but what about all those fancy cappuccinos, mochas, lattes and coffee/cream mixes? Non-diet sodas carry as much as 13 spoons of sugar per can, and fruit juice, though healthy, is high in both calories and sugar.

10 Know Your Cholesterol Levels

You can be fit, lean and healthy and still have a high cholesterol level because of an inherited gene, making you more prone to heart disease. Although only 20% of cholesterol gets there from your diet, it's essential to get your levels checked by your GP.

11 Eat To Sleep Better

Do you find yourself doing embarrassing snores and grunts at night? Research shows that eating more healthy foods and losing weight can cut snoring by 70%, and improve your sleep quality by 40%.

12 Keep A Food Diary For A Week

You'll be surprised at just how much you do eat and when. Most people honestly believe they don't eat much, but add in all those picky foods like nuts, sweets and the odd chip, and you'll see how calories add up.

13 Don't Shop When You're Hungry

Research shows you're more likely to buy fast food, snacks and sugar-based foods.

14 **Ignore The Diet Books**
UK health watchdogs recently looked at 15 of the top-selling diet books and warned – dieters should ignore the advice they give because most of it is wrong, and in some cases it is dangerous.

15 **Choose Not To Eat Rubbish**
As all you're doing is inviting in muscle wasting, weak bones, general lethargy and a whole multitude of age-related diseases such as arteriosclerosis (hardening of the arteries resulting in a stroke), all by the time you're 45.

16 **If You're Desperate, Detox**
Okay, it's too late to eat sensibly and you need to get into that dress – what do you do? Well, for three days (and three days only) do a health detox. This means no coffee, bread, sweet things, cheese, alcohol or pasta and lots of water, vegetables, fruit and the odd jacket potato (without butter). It will give you a flatter stomach, get rid of bloating and detox your system.

17 **Tell The Diet Police To Get Lost**
It's hard enough to eat healthily without well-meaning 'friends' and boyfriends saying, 'You're not supposed to be eating THAT!'

18 **Don't Be A Grazer**
Don't look in the fridge every time you can't think of anything else to do – grazing on the odd biscuit, crisp packet and cold leftovers can add an extra 700 calories to your energy intake a day. Do it every day and you'll pile on weight

19 **Choose Foods That Give You Extra Benefits**
Eat wisely and you'll not only improve your shape but also your looks. Oily fish, for instance, is good for your skin, hair and nails; broccoli promotes healthier skin, and bananas are great for energy.

20 **Think Natural**
Can't even be bothered to think about what you need to eat and buy? Then just pick natural products. Research

shows that those of us who eat more raw and natural produce are happier with our weight and our health.

21 Wait Before Opting For Seconds

It takes 20 minutes for your stomach to register that food is on the way, so wait a while before you dish up seconds.

22 Chew Your Food

Your mum was right – chew every mouthful and you won't eat as much, and you'll digest your food without ending up with a bloated stomach.

23 Eat Your Cake and Enjoy It

Researchers at the University of Hull found it was better for your health to go for guilt-free enjoyment when eating rather than the beat yourself up option.

24 Don't Eat Standing Up

It won't aid digestion and you'll eat faster, more, and feel more stressed about eating.

25 Restrict Low Fat Foods

Remember: low fat isn't low calorie.

chapter 2
The sweaty stuff

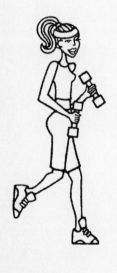

Exercise — why bother?

If you used to hate PE lessons, gymslips and running after a ball at school, you're probably tempted to skip this chapter and, if so, I don't blame you. After all, you already know that you're supposed to exercise and that it's 'good for you' — the problem is (that's if you even think it's a problem) that like over 50% of the population, you can't be bothered.

Maybe you think you're no good it or, like most lazy girls, you imagine you're just not the 'sporty' type, or that gyms are simply an exercise in humiliation! But before you skip this whole chapter, let me just say that the kind of exercise I'm talking about doesn't mean joining a class of ultra-fit Lycra bunnies or doing aerobics five times a week. I'm talking about normal activities you can incorporate into your daily life which, added together, will equal your exercise quota (about five 30-minute sessions a week). If you're still not convinced, here are some reasons why exercise is good for you.

Exercise At Least Three Times A Week And It Will:

- Improve your confidence
- Improve your health
- Improve your sex life
- Help you maintain a weight you're happy with
- Give you healthy skin
- Make you feel happy
- Give you more energy
- Stop you from feeling depressed
- Make you feel strong
- Give you a leaner and fitter body
- Increase your chances of better health when you're older
- Prevent heart disease
- Lower your blood pressure
- Prevent diabetes
- Burn calories
- Slow down the ageing process
- Make you feel more relaxed
- Make you feel more awake
- Make you feel more attractive
- Make you feel anything is possible
- Make you feel you can ring up your old PE teacher and tell her to get stuffed

Top exercise excuses

1. I haven't got time

Studies show most people have at least 45 minutes a day when they could exercise. The problem is that they see exercise as a chore and this 45 minutes as relaxation time, so choose to lie on the couch. The way to do this is not to wait for the day when you have enough money/time/enthusiasm to get to a gym, but to start right now while you're watching TV, walking to work, going shopping, or even cooking your dinner.

If you were feeling especially enthusiastic, you could even get down on the floor right now and do some sit ups as you read this chapter, although that could be going too far. But do bear this simple fact in mind: to clock up 30 minutes of cardiovascular work per day all you have to do is a brisk 15-minute walk to a friend's house and back. And exercise is cumulative. Do it in 10-minute spurts every hour that you're at home (morning and evening), and by the end of the day you should have 50 minutes under your belt.

If you've got 5 minutes to spare . . . climb the stairs. You'll burn off between 100 and 150 calories if you run.

If you've got 10 minutes to spare . . . do a quick fitness circuit. Run on the spot for two minutes, do sit-ups for two minutes, and then run again for one minute. Take a breather for 45 seconds, do press-ups (keep your knees on the floor if you need to) for two minutes, step-ups for two minutes and then stretch for a minute.

If you've got 15 minutes to spare . . . go for a fast walk – this will burn around 100 calories, work your calf muscles, your arms (if you pump them back and forth as you walk), your thighs and – if you pull your stomach in – your lower abdominal muscles.

2. Exercise won't help me to lose weight so what's the point?

While it's very difficult to lose weight just by exercising (to lose half a kilo (1lb) of fat you need to use up 3,500 calories, which would be quite a fantastic feat by exercise alone), doing it alongside healthy eating will:

- Double your weight loss ability and improve your overall health
- Lead to a cumulative effect – walk (at a pace) five times a week for a month and you'll lose well over half a kilo (1lb) of fat (even if you eat the odd cream cake)
- Speed up your metabolism, because toned muscle tissue has a much higher metabolic rate than fat, meaning you will burn more calories and see results quicker

"exercise can completely change the shape of your body."

In addition, while dieting can help you lose fat, exercise can completely change the shape of your body. Fat takes up five times as much space as muscle. So if you replace fat with muscle, your hips, bottom and thighs will be much smaller and leaner. It's also worth remembering that muscle weighs more than fat – so even though you'll be and look smaller, you may weigh only slightly less. Yet another reason to ignore the scales and go by how your clothes feel.

3. What if I start exercising and then stop? Will all my muscle turn to fat?

This one's total nonsense – muscle and fat are different body tissues, so if you stop exercising you won't get fat because of muscle loss, but probably because you're eating too much and not moving.

4. I don't want to lift weights because I'll look like a body builder

Only a very small minority of women are genetically placed to end up looking like a body builder and this is because they have a larger muscle mass than other women. Even then, they have to do masses of exercise, change their diet and lift hefty (as in extremely heavy) weights for at least two hours every day. This regime is unlikely to ever be yours, especially if you're reading this languishing on your sofa.

5. My friend's thighs got really chunky when she started working out

If they did, it's probably because she kept working just one area of her body. Studies show that we're all inclined to exercise the parts of our bodies that are already strong and not vary our routine. If you keep pumping away at something like the step machine because you're good at it, all you'll be doing is working your leg muscles to the extreme and ignoring the muscles that do need to be worked.

6. I don't have the energy or time to work out

Even more reason to work out. Fatigue is a vicious cycle – lie down because you're tired and you'll feel more tired. Forcing yourself to move will actually give you more energy. If you really are exhausted by 6 pm, think about what you're eating. It could be that your breakfast and lunch are depleting your energy levels – help yourself by getting up half an hour earlier and doing some morning exercise, and then go to bed half an hour earlier so you don't miss out on sleep.

The truth about sweating your stuff

The reason why the majority of us don't want to exercise is simply because we are incredibly lazy by nature. But the side effects of being a couch potato are quite huge.

Do No Exercise Whatsoever, And It's Likely You:

- Have gone up a dress size in the past five years
- Get depressed
- Have trouble sleeping
- Feel lethargic
- Lack energy

tips

Exercising three times a week (or two hours a week) could totally change your life.

- Suffer from PMT
- Suffer from post-lunch slumps
- Have backache (caused by weak stomach muscles)

You're Also At A Higher Risk Of:

- Heart disease
- A stroke
- Arthritis
- Osteoporosis

So think about this – instead of a future of aches and pains, just 20–40 minutes of exercise, three times a week (or two hours a week) could totally change your life. To achieve this kind of fitness, you don't have to join an expensive gym, get a personal trainer, run in the park, humiliate yourself in step classes or invest in fancy trainers. All you have to do is get your body moving to the point where you feel a little breathless for only 20 minutes a day. This means you could walk more, have sex more, run on the spot in your flat, or even run up the escalators on the way to work. It will reduce your risk of coronary heart disease by 50%, lower your risk of ovarian, cervical and bowel cancer, and eradicate most of the aches and pains listed above. Here's how to do it:

Step one: move at the right intensity

The aim is to exercise at your 'training' heart rate, which is between 60–75% of your Age Predicted Maximum Heart

Rate (APMHR). It's way too easy to be a lazy exerciser and work out so slowly that you reap no health rewards whatsoever.

You can work out your training heart rate by first taking your age and subtracting it from 220 – this will give you your APMHR – and then calculating 60–75% of that. So if you are 30 years old, your APMHR is 190 and your training heart rate zone is between 114–142.

training zones

Age	AMPHR	60–75%
20	200	120–150
25	195	117–146
30	190	114–142
35	185	111–139

If you can't be bothered to work this one out, the trick is to exercise at an intensity where you feel breathless but can hold a conversation. If you feel you can't breathe, you can't speak, or are going to faint – you're working too hard. Likewise, if you can sing along to MTV and have a chat with the person next to you – you're not working at all.

Step two: do some aerobic exercise

Aerobic exercise isn't jumping up and down for 45 minutes in a class with 20 other women. It's exercise that involves a high level of exertion and so requires a lot of oxygen, breathing and heart-pumping work. Do it regularly and you will be a lean mean fighting machine with energy to burn. This is great if you want to lose weight because it means the more you do the more your body fat will be burnt off. It will also boost your immunity and reduce your risk of a serious illness and heart disease.

The Best Aerobic Exercise:

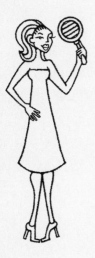

- Walking: improves cardiovascular (the way your lungs and heart work) strength and muscle strength. It's also cheap, easy and can be done in high heels (good for calf strength)
- Swimming: improves upper and lower body muscles as well as aerobic strength. It's also cheap and isn't difficult – but make sure you push yourself and don't just float and glide
- Running: elevates the heart rate and works the lower body – you can do it in local park or in your house up and down the stairs for 20 minutes, or even on the spot
- Cycling: is high quality aerobic exercise that works the arms and legs, and can actually be fun
- Dancing: can burn as many as 500 calories an hour and is easy to fit into your social life
- Do any of the above four to five times a week, for at least 20 minutes each time.

Step three: Add some anaerobic exercise

Anaerobic exercise is exercise that uses muscle strength rather than oxygen, and is also known as strength or weight training. It's good for your fitness levels because it strengthens your bones, tones and shapes your body, and helps you to build up muscles. The women with the best bodies don't do aerobics every day, they lift weights three times a week instead. This is because for each additional kilogram (2lbs) of muscle you build through strength training, you burn 20 to 30 more calories per day. Plus, once you've built muscle mass, you will continue to burn calories even when you're not doing anything.

Regular Anaerobic Exercise Will Help You:

- Feel stronger
- Burn more calories
- Have better muscle tone
- Increase muscle mass, which will keep your body healthy
- Reduce body fat
- Control blood pressure
- Feel better
- Sleep better
- Concentrate better
- Have more energy

The best lazy anaerobic exercise ... is any exercise that increases your muscle strength. It can be any kind of work with weights (lift baked bean cans if you have to), or press ups in front of the TV, tennis, and/or power walking, where you pump your arms as you walk. You need to do it two to three times a week for at least 20 minutes, but not continuously. The best way is to do three sets of 12 repetitions with a break between each set. The aim is to feel the muscles slightly 'burn' on your last two repeats. If you're a beginner, start with eight repetitions and work up to 12.

A lazy guide to getting fitter

Bear in mind that any change will challenge even the laziest body and help you burn more calories. Apart from the obvious connection with weight loss, being active will change a lot of things in your life. If you feel daunted by the whole idea, remember that a little bit of exercise is better for you than none at all. If you can only manage to do something once a week or in 10 minute bursts over the day, that's better than not doing anything.

"a little bit of exercise is better for you than none at all."

Here's how even the laziest girl can get fit:

Identify your fitness personality!

If you want to take up something that you'll stick at, it's obviously better to go for something you'll enjoy and therefore want to do. If you hate moving at all, then you're a lost cause. However, if you have a look around, it's likely you'll eventually find something that matches your personality, and fits in with your daily habits.

According to a 5000-year-old Indian health tradition called Ayurveda, knowing your body type is the key to achieving a great body. Ayurvedic medicine is based around the concept that each body should be treated differently to maximise weight loss, fitness and health. To achieve this, you first have to look at the three governing forces at work in your body, known as vata, pitta and kapha. Each person has a dominant energy, which is set at birth and determines not only physical appearance, but also personality. It may sound like a load of old nonsense, but these body types actually correspond to the traditional Western models of ectomorph (vata), mesomorph (pitta) and endomorph (kapha).

To find out which body type you fall into, answer the following questions, totalling your score after each section. The section in which you score the highest amount of yes's, corresponds to your body type.

(A)

Are you wiry and lean?	Yes/No
Do you have dry skin?	Yes/No
Do you have an erratic memory?	Yes/No
Do you get bored and restless easily?	Yes/No
Do you have a high sex drive?	Yes/No
Do you feel the cold?	Yes/No
Do you prefer hot food?	Yes/No
Do you find it easy to exercise?	Yes/No
Are you energetic?	Yes/No
Total score	4

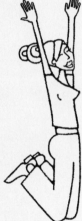
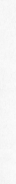

(B)

Are you of medium build?	Yes/No
Do you have smooth skin?	Yes/No
Do you have a good appetite?	Yes/No
Do you have fine hair?	Yes/No
Are you of high intelligence?	Yes/No
Do you never feel too hot or too cold?	Yes/No
Do you prefer cold food?	Yes/No
Are you competitive?	Yes/No
Total score	4

(C)

Are you curvy?	Yes/No
Do you have trouble losing weight?	Yes/No
Do you have thick hair?	Yes/No
Do you have big eyes?	Yes/No
Do you have a happy disposition?	Yes/No

Are you very calm?   Yes/No

Do you feel the hot and the cold?   Yes/No

Do you dislike exercise?   Yes/No

Total score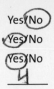

Mostly A – You Are A Vata/Ectomorph

If you are a vata type, it's likely you are slim with long legs and arms. Vata types also tend to be bony and energetic, quick and active. If your energy is off balance, due to a rubbish diet and no exercise, it's likely you will suffer from insomnia and possibly anxiety or panic attacks.

- Go for cardiovascular exercise, which suits your fast-paced nature. However, as you have trouble building muscle mass, you also need to weight train to increase your strength
- Your energy comes in spurts so you need to add in some exercise which is slow and calm. Yoga, ballet, dance aerobics, t'ai chi and gymnastics are all good, as they help relieve stress, control breathing and build up lean muscle mass

Mostly B – You Are A Pitta/Mesomorph

Pittas are of medium build, usually athletic-looking, and have moderate to low body fat. If you are a pitta, you will be strong and muscular. Sturdily built, it's likely you are pear shaped with hips larger than your shoulders, and your legs are the same length as your torso. When your energy is off balance, you are liable to skin complaints, digestive problems and hot flushes.

- As you are usually focused on winning rather than enjoying, team sports do not suit your nature, so do something at your own pace. Try exercise regimes that are about self-control and balance, like Pilates or ballet
- Pittas have the easiest time building up muscle mass, so you need to steer clear of step classes and do exercise that elongates the muscles rather than builds bulk, like yoga

Mostly C – You Are A Kapha/Endomorph

As a kapha, you have a curvy, softer and wider body than pitta or vata types. You're also likely to be of average or short height. Your legs are shorter than your torso, and your breasts tend to be larger than average. If your dosha (energy) is off balance you're likely to suffer from weight gain, lethargy and PMT.

- Kapha types have weaker upper bodies and strong lower bodies. A shorter muscle structure and slow metabolism also means you have a tendency to gain weight around your stomach. You need to focus, therefore, on cross training, swimming, running and weight training. Cross training is particularly good as it will work different parts of the body in different ways, achieving both aerobic and aerobic workouts
- You often have problems with posture as you carry stress in your neck and hold fat in the stomach and hip area. This means you have weak abdominal muscles, which causes stress in the back. In order to strengthen these areas, you

need to firm up all their muscle groups and incorporate stretching into all your workouts

- Less active than the other types, you should choose exercise that involves participation and mutual support. Working with a personal trainer, following a gym programme, or team sports are all ideal

Get motivated

If you still aren't particularly inspired to move your butt, which is probably growing bigger by the second – a by-product of sofa slouching – here's how to help yourself get moving:

- Get an exercise buddy. Either convince a slothful pal to give it a go or push yourself and team up with a gym-mad friend (choose the option that inspires you most)
- Go shopping – not for exercise (though it does count), but because investing in something exercise-related like sexy workout gear means you're more likely to use it
- If nothing else gets you running on the spot, remember that exercise instantly starts burning what you eat, no matter how fattening, greasy or chocolate-smothered

Exercise at home

Too lazy to get to a gym? Make your home a fitness palace.

- Make the bed – taking off sheets, turning the mattress, pulling sheets straight, tucking sheets in, plumping up pillows and duvets can burn off at least 50 calories

- Dig up your garden or mow the lawn. It will use up 150 calories
- Run for the bus – a five-minute sprint will burn around 100 calories
- Do more housework – vacuuming, ironing, dusting and hanging out the washing will each burn about 100 calories
- Have more sex (see Chapter 4 for more details). Thirty minutes of morning sex at a fairly active pace (i.e. get on top) is worth an hour in the afternoon in terms of boosting your metabolic rate and burning fat. This is because the body converts fat stores into energy in the morning. Calories used tot up to 250 per 30-minute session

"exercise instantly starts burning what you eat."

The good thing about exercise is that every little bit counts, so think about doing moves while you go about your everyday business:

- In the shower – do some calf raises (go up and down on your toes, holding for one second and then going down again). This will work your calf muscles and bottom
- Waiting for the bath to fill up – lie face up on the floor with your feet on a chair and do three sets of 12 stomach crunches (put your hands behind your head and curl your head, chest and shoulders forward towards your thighs using your stomach muscles). The trick here is not to yank your head forwards with your hands, but to keep your bottom on the

ground, pull down under your arms and let your tummy do all the work

- On the phone – do some lunges (step forward with one leg, and then drop the knee behind to the floor) and squats (keep both knees directly over the feet and drop your bottom towards the floor). It will work your leg and bottom muscles
- Making tea – do 20 press ups against the wall. You'll exercise your back, triceps, chest and shoulders

You also need to start stretching. It's easily done in front of the TV and just 10 minutes a day will lengthen your muscles, help prevent injury, allow more blood to flow into your brain and help you to feel more relaxed. How to stretch is easy when you know how. Firstly, don't over stretch – if it hurts, stop. Go to where you can in the stretch and breathe into it. Daily stretches to try are:

- Back stretch: stand straight with your feet hip-width apart. Raise your arms above your head (keeping your shoulders down), breathe in and drop your arms and upper body towards the floor, going down as far as you can go. Think about dropping your head towards your knees. Once there, breathe in for two counts and come back up. Repeat five times
- Leg stretch: lie on the floor with your legs straight out in front of you. Now, keeping your bottom and head on the floor, lift one leg straight up (slowly) and place both hands behind the thigh. Now slowly pull the leg towards you. It may not go very far but this will stretch out your hamstring, giving

tips

Have more sex. Thirty minutes of morning sex at a fairly active pace is worth an hour in the afternoon in terms of boosting your metabolic rate and burning fat.

your legs more flexibility and length. Repeat on the other leg
and hold for five counts

- Hip stretch: lie on your back with your arms stretched out to
the side, then bend both legs at the knees with your feet on
the floor. Now roll the knees slowly to the left until they are
on the floor and hold for 10 counts. This will stretch out your
hip and waist. Repeat on the other side for 10 counts

- Arm stretch: lift your left arm above your head (keep the
shoulder down), then bend your arm, and let your hand fall
behind your left shoulder. Place your right hand on the elbow
of your left arm and push down gently. You should feel a
stretch in the back of the left arm. Repeat five times and
change arms

Exercise outside

Too embarrassed to exercise in front of your house mates?
Take it outside . . .

- Get walking. Up your pace and you'll be giving yourself a
moderate work out. The aim is to do it for 20 minutes and
feel a bit breathless while you're doing it. Do it in high heels
and you'll give your calves an extra workout. Do it with heavy
shopping bags on each arm and you'll give your arm muscles
a boost. Help yourself by playing something loud on your
walkman to boost your energy. Afterwards make sure you
stretch or else you'll have sore calves

- Climb more stairs (and don't take the lift). If you can spare only 10 minutes a day to exercise, climbing or running up and down stairs is the most challenging way to exercise. It will give you a fantastic cardiovascular workout, costs nothing and works your entire body

Exercise at your office

Avoid work boredom and improve your muscle tone.

tips

Walk everywhere. It will give you a fantastic cardio-vascular workout, costs nothing and works your entire body.

- Work your abdominal muscles at your desk by sitting up straight with your feet on the ground. Now breathe in, and on the out breath, pull your belly button and lower abs into the back of your spine as far as you can and hold for 10 seconds, breathing at the same time. Release and repeat 12 times. Do this for five minutes, five times a day, and you'll have strong abdominals in no time (and these are better than sit ups)

- Multitask. If you really can't be bothered to spend 40 minutes a day on exercise (20 on cardio, 20 on weights and stretching), then multitask. Running up and down the stairs with heavy shopping bags, work files or boxes should do the trick

- Squeeze your bum. While waiting for the kettle to boil or the photocopier, squeeze your bottom cheeks together really hard for 10 seconds. Do this five times a day and you'll notice a difference in two weeks. This is because the muscles in the bottom will hold in a semi-flexed position for up to 20 minutes afterwards, working the muscle and lifting your bum

25 reasons to move your butt

1 You're Better At It Than Men

The majority of women fare better in the fitness arena than men, thanks mainly to lifestyle choices. Having said this, being female means you can expect to gain on average almost 5 kg (11lb) between the ages of 35 and 45, and to start losing 1% of bone mass a year after menopause. But it doesn't take much to reverse these scary stats. A recent study in the *Journal of the American Medical Association* showed that exercising (cardio and strength training) just three times a week for a year can decrease the age of your body by 10–15 years.

2 It Has Long-term Benefits

Researchers estimate that for every hour of exercise you take, you increase your life expectancy by two hours. Plus, exercise stimulates the growth of new brain cells (particularly helpful if you've been destroying them with alcohol), and lowers your risk of Alzheimer's disease.

3 It Will Make You Happy

A new study from the University of New York medical school has discovered that exercise is better medicine than medicine itself. The study compared people on antidepressants to people taking exercise and found that those who regularly worked out showed greater improvement than those who didn't. This is because raising your heart rate through exercise increases serotonin levels in the brain in much the same way that antidepressants do.

4 It Will Help You To Stand Up Straight

Slouching may be comfy but standing up burns twice as many calories as sitting down. Plus, if you stand up straight, pull your shoulders down, and stomach in, you'll look taller, leaner and be working your muscles all in one go.

5 It Will Lower Your Blood Pressure

Blood pressure is the force exerted by your blood against the walls of your arteries. If your blood pressure is too high it can kill you, and it's also a major cause of strokes and heart attacks. Luckily, blood pressure can be lowered for good with regular exercise.

6 It Will Lower Your Cholesterol Levels

Exercise greatly reduces harmful cholesterol, which is a good thing because this fat deposit on the linings of the artery walls ups your chances of a heart attack.

7 It Will Strengthen Your Bones

It takes just 20 minutes of cardiovascular and weight-bearing exercise, e.g. jogging, walking and lifting weights, three times a week to strengthen your bones. American studies have now shown that walking a mile a day also reduces the risk of osteoporosis (brittle bones) in later life.

8 It Will Stop You Gaining Weight

By the time you reach your 30s you start losing muscle mass and have more fat in your body, which is why you can get away with being a couch potato when you're young but not when you're older. However, if you keep exercising you'll retain your muscle for longer.

9 It Will Improve Your Skin

Pumping blood round your body is a natural skin booster. If you want an instant radiant glow that lasts all day, exercise three to five times a week.

10 It Will Keep You Looking Sexy

Regular exercise will delay your body's natural degeneration and keep your body fit and able. Meaning, you won't be hunched over and wheelchair-bound by the time you're 70.

11 It Will Improve Your Self-esteem

Feeling stronger will help you to feel better about your body and your mind.

12 It Will Stop PMS

Exercise can relieve PMS by releasing feel-good chemicals into the bloodstream. It also eases the physical PMS symptoms of bloating and headaches, and lessens pre-period pain.

13 It Will Boost Your Fertility

Plus it makes labour easier, gives you a healthier baby, and a better chance of getting pregnant when you want.

14 It Will Lower Your Risk Of Breast Cancer

Breast cancer currently affects 1 in 12 women in the UK, yet studies show that if you exercise regularly you can lower your risk by nearly 60%.

15 It Will Boost Your Energy

Exercising boosts your breathing capacity, which means you take in more oxygen, which means better circulation and better energy levels.

16 It Will Help You Sleep Better

Just a simple half-an-hour walk a day can relax you and make you sleep more easily because exercise uses up excess adrenaline in the body. Regular exercise can beat insomnia and reduce snoring.

17 It Will Keep You Warmer

Always cold? If you exercise you'll tune your internal boiler and won't need to sit shivering through the winter. Research shows that exercisers use their body heat more effectively than non-exercisers.

18 It Will Lower Your Stress Levels

Because exercise fights off the chemicals released by stress in the body and replaces them with feel-good hormones. It also releases tension in your muscles and helps you relax.

19 It Will Improve Your Relationships

Exercise is a mood booster. If you're happy you're less likely to argue with or pick on your boyfriend or workmates.

20 It Will Improve The Big O

Studies show that exercisers have better orgasms and higher arousal levels than couch potatoes. It's all down to the increased blood flow to the genital area and a fitter heart rate.

21 It Will Get Rid Of Your Backache

It's estimated that over 50% of people suffer from back complaints. If you're already feeling twinges, the chances are you have weak stomach muscles and your back is having to support both your front and behind. You can improve the situation by incorporating strength-building abdominal exercises into your exercise programme.

22 You Will Stay Healthier For Longer

Exercise is vital for the prevention of disease and infections. It boosts the immune system and stimulates the body to fight off new infections.

23 It Will Improve Your Brain

Studies also show that exercise can even make you smarter by boosting brain activity.

24 It Will Help You To Stay Away From Bad Habits

A recent study has shown that exercise makes you twice as likely to stick to a weight loss programme, and twice as likely to be successful at giving up smoking.

25 You Will Feel The Benefits Instantly

The instant you start to exercise you'll feel better. Just one walk can decrease feelings of hopelessness, boost optimism and lower anxiety.

chapter 3
Horrible habits

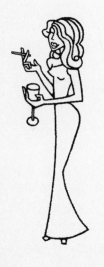

Are bad habits bad for your health?

Smoking, drinking, partying, late nights and caffeine-fuelled mornings – bad for your health? Definitely! Will that make you stop? I doubt it. The fact is that when it comes to certain habits, no amount of government health warnings will stop a lazy girl having a good time.

If this sounds like your life, I won't bother to tell you the obvious because, like me, you already know that smoking will kill you, hangovers are signs you have poisoned yourself and caffeine is not a food group. I will suggest, however, that even the wildest party girl can benefit from reassessing her horrible habits. While I'm not advocating a total life change, it's would be well worth interjecting some healthy parts into your unhealthy bits, especially if you want to live a long and relatively healthy life.

Step one is to get your facts straight about what you're really doing to yourself. Step two is to look at ways you can avoid those nasty morning-after moments and still fuel your hedonistic nights, and step three is to stop fooling yourself that you're being healthy when you obviously aren't. Here's all you'll ever need to know about your horrible habits.

Boozing

It's the weekend, you've had a stressful day, it's someone's birthday, you've got a new boyfriend, you're boyfriend-less – oh, any old excuse for a quick one down the pub. For 97% of the population, alcohol is a mainstay of socialising – a way of relaxing, unwinding and avoiding the stress of everyday life. It does no harm, does it? What's more, you've probably read a tipple is good for you. But the health benefits of alcohol are not what they are cracked up to be. While a glass of red wine a night has been proven to be good for your heart, more than two and you'll start damaging your liver, dehydrating your skin and killing off some much needed brain cells.

Here's what alcohol can do to your body:

Make your bones brittle
Alcohol and osteoporosis (the bone crumbling disease) are linked because drinking accelerates the loss of nutrients from the body, meaning your bones lose out.

Raise your blood pressure
Drinking anything more than small amounts, even just a couple of drinks after work, can raise your blood pressure. If you booze it up regularly your blood pressure levels can stay high and won't improve until you cut back.

Give you heartburn
Alcohol is very acidic and gulping large amounts can cause a nasty burning sensation in your chest and throat, making it hard to swallow, and bringing up some nasty bile into your throat.

Aggravate PMS
Women who drink a lot are more prone to PMS symptoms because of the high sugar content in alcohol. This upsets your blood sugar levels and robs you of the nutrients you need to beat PMS.

Ruin your skin
Alcohol can make you look older because booze dehydrates

you and decreases the elasticity of the skin, causing it to age faster, get more wrinkled and basically make you look like an old hag.

Make you miserable

Well, it might make you happy for a few hours but the truth is, alcohol is a depressant, which means it takes you to a nice rosy high and then brings you crashing back down to earth and brings on the blues.

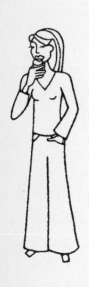

Pickle your liver

Also known as cirrhosis, liver pickling occurs when liver cells die and the liver tissue starts to scar. It's a direct result of long-term daily drinking, so if you have been boozing most days since your 21st birthday it's time to give it a break. Thankfully, the liver can repair itself, but only if you give it time to do so.

What happens when you drink

You may feel elated, euphoric and super-confident after a few glasses of wine but these feelings are an illusion. Alcohol has this effect because it turns off the part of the brain that controls your judgement. This means your normal inhibitions (safety switches that stop you dancing naked on tabletops) disappear. Hence the common morning-after refrain, 'Oh my god, did I really do that?'.

Sadly, studies the world over show that drinking regularly or indulging in weekend binges, ups your chances of having a one-night stand, risking unprotected sex, eating badly and making large errors of judgement that can cause dangerous accidents.

Part of the problem is that, unlike food, alcohol is absorbed directly into the bloodstream, and stays swilling around your body until the liver burns it up. This happens slowly, at the rate of one unit an hour – so if you drink five vodkas and two glasses of wine, you'll stay intoxicated for a further seven hours. As a female, alcohol also affects the body in more dangerous ways. For a start, we get drunk quicker than men who weigh the same as us because we have fewer of the enzymes in the liver that help break down alcohol. Also female bodies have 10% more body fat (a genetic fact so don't panic) and less water than male ones, which means we can't handle our alcohol as well as men can.

Just Three Drinks In One Night Will:

- Reduce your chance of having a decent orgasm. Booze lowers your arousal levels and anaesthetises you, so you feel less
- Give you more body fat. Three large glasses of wine and then chips/pizza/kebabs on the way home can add 0.25 kg (^{1}/2 lb) of fat to your body. This is because your body will burn off useless calories first (the alcohol ones) and store the rest as fat

tips

The weekly alcohol limit for women is 14 units. Units apply to pub measures so if you are drinking at home, you are probably getting through more units than you think.

- Fur up your arteries, because alcohol increases levels of bad fats called triglycerides in the blood
- Give you weak bones – by slowing down the bone building cells in the body
- Give you blurry vision. Alcohol paralyses the eye muscles, meaning you can't focus and can't work out distances properly. It also interferes with co-ordination in the brain, which means you're more likely to fall down
- Give you stomach problems, because alcohol can inflame and ulcerate the lining of the digestive tract
- Poison sperm and damage ovum, making conception difficult
- Contribute towards cardiovascular disease, putting you at a higher risk of heart disease

Know your limits

You probably already know that the weekly alcohol limit (for a woman) is 14 units, but this is a standard – meaning it may be too high for you. If you are smaller and weigh less you will get drunk quicker and faster than someone who is bigger than you. Plus, units apply to pub measures. If you are drinking at home, you are probably getting through more units than you think. Remember, a unit equals half a pint of normal strength beer, a small glass of wine, or a standard measure of spirits.

The lazy girl's guide to safer drinking

- Eat before you start drinking – you'll drink less
- Don't order double measures
- Aim to drink no more than one alcoholic drink an hour
- Have a soft drink in between each measure of alcohol
- Add a mixer to your drink to dilute it
- Watch your measures at home
- Avoid cocktails – there can be three units in one glass. Plus, if you drink your booze through a straw you'll get drunk faster as you will consume more alcohol than a usual gulp.
- Read the alcohol percentage strength on beer bottles – a strong beer equals two units
- Don't be fooled by alcoholic soft drinks – a quarter of a pint of alcoholic lemonade is one unit
- After-dinner liqueurs count as units
- Fizzy alcohol like champagne will get you drunk faster because the bubbles speed the alcohol into your bloodstream
- Drink slower – it will give your body more time to deal with the alcohol

Drinking myths

Myth: *You don't drink too much because you never get hangovers*

If you can pack away 10 units without getting drunk, it

"hangovers are a sign that you have poisoned yourself."

doesn't mean your body can handle alcohol better than most. It's more likely you've become used to handling large amounts of alcohol which, let's face it, is not a good sign!

Myth: *You won't gain weight because you never eat when you drink*
Opt for alcohol over food in a bid to keep weight off and you're wasting your time. Three pints of beers and you've drunk 600 calories, which could have been a full meal, plus the energy value will be useless because you won't be gaining any nutrients, just plain calories.

Myth: *You only drink at weekends so it's okay*
Binge drinking has been shown to be just as bad for your health as daily drinking. Weekend bingers consume more drink in one night that most people do in a whole week, which makes the effects more damaging, and alcohol poisoning more likely.

Myth: *Alcohol is good for you*
While studies may show that one drink a day is good for your heart and ups levels of what is known as good cholesterol (HDL), the protective effects stop as soon as you drink more than two drinks. Take a look on the next page:

The lowdown on four of your favourite tipples

red wine	While red wine provides potassium, iron and various antioxidants, it also contains a compound called tyramine, which can induce a killer hangover and headache
lager	Contains antioxidants, magnesium, folic acid and B vitamins, but also nearly 200 calories a pint, so not good for your waistline
gin and tonic	Low in chemicals because it's a pure spirit, but devoid of any minerals or vitamins
Bailey's	Chocolate-tasting alcohol which contains as much fat as two chocolate biscuits, and that's if you stick to a small measure

Myth: *You're not an alcoholic, so what's the worry?*
Being a problem drinker and having a problem with drinking are two different things. If you wake up more than once a week with a hangover, regularly throw sickies to recover from the night before and generally have alcohol induced depressions – you have a problem with your booze that needs sorting.

Myth: *You're safe because you never mix your drinks*
While mixing the grape and the grain will give you a nasty headache due to the congeners (chemicals found in alcohol

which irritate the brain) in beer and wine, there's no evidence that this makes you drunk quicker. The only reason mixing results in a hangover is that you are more likely to drink more units.

Beating your hangovers the lazy way

We've all been there – the spinning room, the thumping headache and the rising nausea – yes, it's the hangover from hell and it's happening to you. And it's happening because, thanks to last night, there are now vast quantities of alcohol, chemicals and nasties swimming around your body. You feel nauseous because your blood sugar levels have gone haywire and the acid in the alcohol is irritating your stomach. Headaches occur for two reasons: one – you're dehydrated because the alcohol in your body has been acting like a diuretic all night and tricked your body into peeing too much; two – drinks like red wine and whisky switch on the brain's pain receptors causing that nasty stabbing behind your eyes. You feel weak because high levels of insulin have been produced as a response to all that sugar you've taken in – you probably also feel faint and hungry. You feel tired because alcohol interferes with REM sleep, meaning you will wake up feeling as if you haven't slept at all.

Luckily you can avoid all this by doing the following:

1. Don't drink on an empty stomach

The advice your mother gave you is true: a full stomach slows down alcohol absorption. Good foods to eat are ones that are easily digested. Toast, a sandwich, pasta and yoghurt all protect the stomach lining. Foods that are processed or high in sugar will only take the alcohol with them into the bloodstream.

2. Take some supplements

Antioxidants are particularly good at fighting off alcohol damage and protecting your liver. They also stop your brain cells being killed off by weekend binges. Found in green leafy vegetables and fruit. Also aim to get ample amounts of vitamins A, C and E in the days before a big night out as this is used up in huge amounts to break down alcohol in the body.

3. Drink plenty of water

Before you go to sleep make yourself drink a pint of water to stop dehydration. It will also help rid your body of the toxin acetaldehyde, which is released by the liver when alcohol is broken down. (It is this toxin that causes dehydration and leads to a thumping head.) Water and fruit juice the morning after will also help balance your blood sugar levels and re-hydrate you.

4. Eat something healthy the morning after

You may be craving a fry-up for comfort reasons and to assuage your hunger, but cramming all that fat into your body will just make you feel ill an hour after your meal. Your aim should be to

tips

After a heavy night out, drink a pint of water to stop de-hydration. Water in the morning will also help re-hydrate you.

stabilise your blood sugar, so you need to eat small portions frequently. Think about fruit juice, toast and honey, porridge or cereal.

5. Take some medication

Painkillers taken with food can help your headache, but don't take any before you go to sleep because alcohol levels will be too high in your body. Take them alone and you'll be irritating your stomach lining. Also, think about taking a herbal supplement before you go to sleep and when you wake up. Both milk thistle and artichoke have been shown to help protect the liver from alcohol damage and reduce hangovers by speeding up the breakdown of alcohol in the body.

6. Drink something disgusting – the Prairie Oyster

A raw egg swallowed whole (no oyster involved – the name comes from the slang for a bull's testicle) supposedly works due to a chemical found in eggs known as cysteine, which helps metabolise alcohol.

7. Sip a fizzy diet drink

Another cure for feeling sick is to drink flat cola. It's said to settle the stomach and ease nausea. Fizzy diet drinks can also help settle the stomach, but avoid non-diet ones as the sugar will further upset your blood sugar levels.

8. Be honest about why you always have hangovers

Can't have fun without alcohol? Are you sure, or is it that you've forgotten how to actually have fun without a drink or two (or ten)? Bear in mind that the best way to have fun the day after being out is to not overdo it the night before. If you're supposedly boozing for social reasons, be honest and don't lie to yourself. Will your friends really know if your tonic has gin in it? Will they really be disappointed if you dilute your wine with water?

9. Give yourself time to get over it

The best cure in the world is to rest up and avoid alcohol for a few days. You'll give your body a chance to jettison the excess alcohol swilling around your gut. Eat healthily and give yourself a decent night's sleep, and the morning after 'the morning after' you'll feel fine.

These two, on the other hand, won't do you any good at all:

1. Hair of the dog, i.e. more drink

Totally useless. It might reduce short-term hangover symptoms, but the result is temporary.

2. Black coffee

This might make you feel more alert but it won't help get rid of alcohol in the body, and will only aid dehydration by making you pee more, add to your thumping headache and irritate your stomach lining. Better to drink water or juice.

Smoking — puffing your way to bad health

We all know smoking kills and that smoking-related diseases are on the increase. The scary bits aside, were you also aware that smoking ages you, gives you bad breath, deep facial lines, dehydrates your skin and makes your periods more painful? All thanks to the 4,000 chemicals a single cigarette holds within its grasp.

Each Cigarette Contains:

- Carbon monoxide – the very same gas found in smelly car exhausts
- Nicotine – a powerful poison that can kill in its natural undiluted state. Also used as a powerful insecticide
- Ammonia – also used to clean kitchen floors!
- Butane – the gas found in cigarette lighters
- Tar – that nice black stuff – 70% of which is deposited over a smoker's lungs

Here's what else smoking will do for you:

Make your sex life more painful

Yes, believe it or not, smoking can short-circuit your pleasure wiring. Female smokers complain of vaginal dryness and painful intercourse more frequently than non-smokers. This is because smoking restricts blood *"ten per cent of female smokers have no orgasms at all."*

flow, which is essential for arousal, and halts lubrication, which is necessary for non-painful sex. If your boyfriend smokes too, he is damaging the arteries that transport the blood necessary for an erection – eventually he's going to have problems getting it up.

Dampen down your orgasms

Smoking also interferes with your orgasm by limiting clitoral sensitivity: 10% of female smokers have no orgasms at all and 13% have muted ones.

Make contraception choices difficult

Women who smoke are advised not to use the contraceptive pill (or at least to use one with a very low dosage). The hormones in the pill when combined with the chemicals in a cigarette increase your chances of heart disease, making your risk 30 times higher than that of a non-smoker.

Ruin your baby chances

Even though two out of three women quit as soon as they find out they are pregnant, smoking could well stop you even getting to that stage. Cigarette smoke has been shown to decrease fertility levels by as much as 50%. This is because couples who smoke have high levels of cadmium, a heavy toxic metal that stops zinc (essential for fertility), from being absorbed into the body.

Make your skin wrinkly

To stay young and healthy your skin relies on a healthy blood supply pumping away beneath the skin. Nicotine, unfortunately, constricts blood vessels, so starving the skin of vital oxygen.

Give you bad breath

Smoking dries out the membranes inside your mouth that are responsible for producing saliva. With no saliva to regularly kill off bacteria, you're asking for some deadly halitosis. The truth is that most smokers have bad breath (even if they suck extra strong mints), because every puff they take contains chemicals that linger in their mouth and produce some very pungent and nasty smells.

Kill your mega-watt smile

Studies show that smoking can give you gum disease. Gingivitis – also known as inflammation of the gums – sets in because smoking has eaten away at the mouth's defence mechanism.

Give you chronic bronchitis

Not just a smoker's cough, but a condition that restricts

your air passages and destroys lung tissue. By the time you feel breathlessness, the damage has been done – 30,000 people die in the UK every year from this disease.

Give you a nice wheezy sound

Emphysema is a progressively disabling condition in which the alveoli (air sacs in the lungs) are gradually destroyed, making it difficult to breathe without wheezing. It accounts for one fifth of all smoking-related deaths.

> *"smoking causes one third of all cancer deaths in the UK."*

Make you snore like a pig

Smoking irritates membranes in the nose and throat and causes mucus secretion. At the same time, it turns up the snoring volume by causing the tissues in the nose to swell.

Up your risk of cancer

Smoking causes one third of all cancer deaths in the UK. Put another way, you are 25 times more likely to get lung cancer if you smoke 10 cigarettes or more a day. This is because cigarette smoke is carcinogenic: it increases the risk of cancer in anything it touches – your mouth, your throat, your lungs, even your lips!

Put you at risk of a heart attack

Smoking more than 20 a day brings with it a six times higher heart attack risk. This is because the chemicals in tobacco smoke cause the coronary arteries to constrict, leading to chest pain and chronic arterial damage. The two biggest contributors to heart disease – carbon monoxide and nicotine – are both found in cigarette smoke.

Smoking myths

Myth: *It helps you control your weight*

Weight studies show that women who smoke are only half a kilogram (1lb) thinner than women who don't. As for the idea that if you give up you'll pile it on – in a recent study by Quitline, only 6% of those who had stopped smoking gained weight.

Myth: *You're not addicted*

No, of course not. You could stop any time you wanted to, couldn't you? You're only smoking now because you feel like it. You never crave one when you're having a coffee break/a quick one down the pub/after dinner/when you wake up/after sex – do you? That's okay then!

Myth: *It's legal so it can't be that bad*

Untrue – hence the government health warnings on the side of packs. Cigarettes are legal for lots of reasons, the main one being tax revenue. The UK government makes over £8 billion a year from tobacco sales ($48 billion in the US).

Myth: *It's a stress reliever*

While smoking does have a mild narcotic effect, i.e. it makes you feel sleepy, it's also a powerful stimulant. If you're stressed, all it will do is raise your blood sugar levels and boost adrenaline in the body, adding anxiety and tension to your stress levels.

Myth: *Low tar is better for you*

Actually, no. Studies show that there is no reduction in the risk of having a smoking-related disease from smoking low tar cigarettes.

Myth: *You know someone who smoked all his or her life without any health problems, so it can't be that bad*

And there's probably someone out there who can run across motorways without being knocked over. The fact is that smoking is the largest cause of preventable cancer deaths in Britain. It causes 43,000 deaths a year.

kicking that butt the lazy way

give up and within . . .

20 minutes	your blood pressure will fall
8 hours	the levels of poisonous carbon monoxide in your blood will drop to normal
2 days	your chances of a heart attack will decrease and your sense of smell will start to return

give up and within . . .

3 days	your lung airways will start to relax
2 weeks	your circulation will improve
1 month	your sinus congestion and fatigue will decrease
2 months	your lung function will start to improve
6 months	your overall energy will increase
1 year	premature wrinkling will decrease and your risk of coronary heart disease will drop to half of that of a smoker
3–5 years	your risk of lung cancer will return to normal
10 years	your health risks will drop to the same as for a non-smoker

Reasons To Quit:

- You'll have more money
- You'll have more energy
- You won't pass out walking up the stairs
- You'll smell better
- You'll look better
- You'll have sweet breath
- More people will want to kiss you
- Your family will stop moaning at you
- You won't die prematurely

How To Give Up:

- Decide on a quit date. And before you hit it, make a plan. Detail how you're going to deal with temptation and what your weak spots are. Also, focus on getting through each hour and each day, not on how you're going to cope with the rest of your life without cigarettes

- See your doctor for some advice. If you can, do it without patches or medication. Your doctor may still have some advice on alternative help such as hypnotherapy or acupuncture

- Motivate yourself. Promise yourself a treat for every day that you keep off cigarettes, and a bigger one at the end of six months

- Believe you can do it. Because you can. Smokers become non-smokers every day

- Keep at it. Don't give up just because you slip up. So, you've had one cigarette after your quit date – don't use it as an excuse to start smoking again

- Don't let stress get you down. The stress of not smoking is part of the withdrawal tension from giving up a drug you are addicted to; it's not a reason to start again

- Be aware of what's happening to your body. Nicotine levels in the blood drop every two hours, which is why you become twitchy for a cigarette – be ready to combat that. Withdrawal symptoms only last 3–4 weeks. After that you won't feel so irritated and stressed. As for cravings, these also lessen, though be aware that the urge can suddenly return at stressful moments in your life

tips

Motivate yourself. Promise yourself a treat for every day that you keep off cigarettes, and a bigger one at the end of six months.

- Drink lots of water. It will flush out the toxins hanging about in your body
- Avoid situations where you used to smoke. This will keep temptation at bay until your withdrawal symptoms have passed
- If you fail, try again. On average people try about three times to give up before they manage it for good

If you really can't do it on your own, consider one of the following:

1. Nicotine patches

It's not the nicotine in cigarettes that damages your health but the poisonous chemicals in the tobacco. Nicotine is what keeps you addicted. If you want to give up, patches are good because they administer the nicotine you crave but without the smoking part. The idea is to use them for three months and slowly reduce the patches you use. The good news is that they work, the bad news is that they won't beat your addiction and you still have to work at quitting.

2. Nicotine inhalers

These are plastic, cigarette-shaped objects that are good for people who miss the sucking action of smoking. A nicotine capsule is fitted inside and it delivers a blast of nicotine every time you puff. Again, they work, but won't stop your addiction.

3. Zyban

Available only on prescription under strict guidelines, the drug

Zyban reduces nicotine craving and makes withdrawal easier. The downside is that it comes with a variety of side effects.

4. Alternative therapies

Acupuncture and hypnotherapy are both used frequently by people trying to give up but their effectiveness is still unproven. Hypnosis works by changing subconscious beliefs about quitting and being a smoker. Acupuncture works by stimulating the brain to make withdrawal easier.

Coffee

One minute we're told caffeine is good for us, the next it's the devil's brew. The truth is:

- You can get addicted to it
- You can get withdrawal symptoms from it
- It disturbs your sleep patterns
- It lowers fertility
- It makes you anxious
- It gives you mood swings
- It makes you feel dizzy
- It can upset your stomach
- It gives you headaches
- It aggravates irritable bowel syndrome
- It makes jet-lag worse

Caffeine, believe it or not, is the most widely used drug

around. It's found in coffee, tea, chocolate, soft drinks, cola drinks and fizzy drinks, and we love it because it's a physical and mental stimulant. Have the right amount and even the laziest girl will feel alert and wide-eyed. But drinking too much will make you feel tired, anxious and jittery. Keep drinking, and you can add nervousness, palpitations and insomnia to the mix. Do this repeatedly every day, and you'll have headaches, nausea, diarrhoea, high blood pressure and pretty bad PMS.

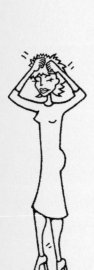

The above happens because caffeine has a chemical effect on your body that mimics the 'fight or flight' stress response (see Chapter 6), which is why more than four cups of coffee will double your stress levels. Experts advise a maximum of 300 mg of coffee a day, but just a normal cup of ground coffee contains around 150 mg. Have a cup at breakfast, one at 11 am and one after lunch and you're already scoring 450 mg, and that's if you've stuck to a medium sized mug!

Kicking the latte habit the lazy way

- Cut down slowly and don't go cold turkey. Caffeine is a drug – cut it out all at once and you're asking for nasty withdrawal symptoms. Set a deadline each day, e.g. no coffee after 2 pm, and then start limiting your intake (and cup size) in the morning

- Go decaf or caffeine-free (this type of cola really does taste the same). It's not as exciting in terms of buzz, but it does help to cut down your caffeine habit
- Don't just replace one caffeine buzz for another – drink more water instead. It will help flush out the coffee you've drunk and re-hydrate you (coffee is a diuretic)
- Be aware of what caffeine does to your body. Coffee contains a chemical called methylxanthine which aggravates your hormones and the way your body functions
- If you're going to drink lots of it, make sure you take a multivitamin and mineral supplement because caffeine interferes with the absorption of calcium, magnesium, zinc and iron

Recreational drugs

Just say no, right? Well, many people just say yes, and – no surprises here – drug use and glowing health don't go hand in hand. Take a look at the following:

1. Ecstasy – also known as E, MDMA and XTC

Basically a stimulant and a hallucinogenic that comes in tablet form. It's no longer sold in a pure state so it's often mixed with LSD, speed and even talcum powder – so beware! Ecstasy works by boosting your energy and increasing your blood pressure and temperature. It's bad news for your health because it stimulates the nervous system so that you can't tell when you're exhausted. If you then forget to drink water continuously you could become seriously ill from dehydration. Side effects also include depression, exhaustion and anxiety attacks.

2. Cannabis (marijuana)

Like many drugs, cannabis has been used for centuries and has medicinal properties – but this doesn't mean it's healthy. While cannabis makes you feel more relaxed and calm, the bad news is that if (like most people) you smoke it and mix it with tobacco, you're inhaling more muck than you usually would from a cigarette. Smoke cannabis every day and you're asking to be in a perpetual dreamlike state in which you can't concentrate, remember things or get by without having another puff.

3. Cocaine

The effects of cocaine only last 30 minutes, which means more and more has to be sniffed in order to keep the effects going. It works by being absorbed into the bloodstream through thin membranes in the nose, and gives an almost immediate energy high. Sadly it can also cause paranoia, anxiety and aggression. Frequent use causes insomnia, depression and destruction of the membranes in the nose.

4. Speed (amphetamines)

A stimulant just like caffeine but much stronger. It will keep you up, keep you going and drive you mad. You'll feel exhilarated for hours on speed, but then won't be able to climb back down and take a much-needed rest. This leads to anxiety, depression, fatigue and dehydration. Do it regularly and you'll feel panic ridden and find yourself with bad skin and a low immune system.

Kicking the drug habit the lazy way

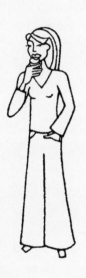

- Seek professional help if you can't give up. Your GP can help, as can the National Drugs Helpline (see Resources)
- Don't mix drugs and alcohol – partly because alcohol further dehydrates your body, but also because the two do not mix well and could lead to a visit to casualty at 2 am
- Go easy on quantities – stacking is a big problem with certain drugs such as ecstasy and speed. The more you take the drug, the more you need in order to achieve the same effect, and so you pile them up – this is a good way to end up overdosing
- Think about your size. As with alcohol, the effect on your body is partly determined by how big you are. If you're 1.5 m tall (5 ft) and weigh 44 kg (7 stones), drugs will hit your bloodstream faster and knock you out quicker
- Never take drugs on your own – there's no one to seek help if you pass out or have a seizure
- Think about why you're using drugs: what it gives you and what it takes away
- Watch out for long-term effects – panic attacks, anxiety, insomnia and depression that won't go away are all signs that you need to think about your health

25 *ways* to deal with horrible habits

1 Indulge Less

The truth is, you can drink yourself young and you can drink yourself old. The difference is slim – have one or two small drinks a day and you'll live slightly longer, have three or more large drinks and you'll age and die faster. The same goes for most bad habits.

2 Drink More Water

It will flush out a variety of toxins from your body and help you at least stay vaguely healthy. Remember: for every pint of beer you drink, your body loses one and a half pints of liquid.

3 Sleep For Longer

Most people need eight hours sleep a night. Get one hour less a night for seven days in a row and by the end of the week you'll have lost a whole night's sleep.

4 Change Your Attitude

You are not born a smoker/drinker/party animal. If you want to stop you can – all it takes is a small change of attitude.

5 Use Some Commonsense

An after-dinner expresso will keep you awake all night. Smoking 10 cigarettes in two hours will give you a hacking great cough, and drinking until you fall over will make you feel like death in the morning.

6 Think About How Much Is Right For You

Be sensible; don't gauge your drinking just by your units – stop when you know you've had enough. Warning signs include dizziness, lack of concentration, that spacey feeling and falling over.

7 Think About What You're Doing

The trouble with habits is that most of us only think about what we've done in hindsight. It sounds dull, but if you're always griping about feeling tired, it's time to think about what you're doing to your body every night.

8 Remind Yourself That You Don't Have To Give It All Up

Studies have shown that people who drink 1–2 units a night have a 30% lower risk of heart disease than teetotallers. So you don't have to become a nun about your habits.

9 Give It Up For Your Baby

You already know smoking can hinder your fertility, but it can also make your life a misery when you're pregnant.

10 Think About Your Sex Life

Studies show that smokers and heavy drinkers enjoy fewer affectionate moments. Apparently, women who smoke give and receive about half as many kisses and hugs as non-smoking women.

11 Think About Your Relationship

Heavy drinkers are twice as likely to end up in the divorce courts, due to more drink-fuelled fights and irritable morning afters.

12 Drink Red Wine

Doctors recommend a glass or two every day to protect the heart. The magic ingredients are polyphenols, which help stop arteries becoming furry and prone to heart disease.

13 Remember That Your Habits Can Kill You

Not just in the future, but right now. Nearly 4,000 UK people a year die from alcohol poisoning and related liver diseases.

14 Avoid Panic Attacks

Studies show you're more likely to have a panic attack within 6 to 12 hours of drinking, and be more prone to them if you are over tired.

15 Think Before You Party Too Hard

Hundreds of brain cells are killed off by weekend drinking binges, but you can help yourself by taking an antioxidant such as vitamin E.

16 Consider Your Kidneys

Alcohol, fizzy drinks, caffeine and citrus juices all irritate the bladder. Give your kidneys a well-deserved break and avoid or cut down on all of these in favour of water.

17 Work Out After A Night Out

It may be the last thing on your mind, but a light morning-after-the-night-before workout will accelerate the body's process of expelling the nasty toxins that are floating around your bloodstream.

18 Detox

If you regularly live it up and know you smoke, drink and eat too much junk, think about a weekend detox to rid you of all the nasties. The principles are simple – avoid all fatty foods and only eat raw vegetables and fruit.

19 Eat More Fruit

Especially after a heavy weekend indulging your bad habits. Apples will cleanse your gut, grapes will aid digestion and pineapple and bananas will restore your blood sugar levels and make you feel cleansed.

20 Don't Drink On An Empty Stomach

Eating won't stop you getting drunk, but it will slow down the process, and stop you getting drunk too fast.

21 Beware Fizzy Drinks

Alcoholic fizzy drinks make you drunk quicker and a can of cola contains roughly the same amount of caffeine as a cup of coffee. What's more, diet and sport fizzy drinks contain more caffeine than standard colas, which is why they can promise a 'lift'.

22 Be Kind To Your Brain

Can't remember what you're supposing to be doing? It's not lack of concentration, but the result of too much caffeine and alcohol, say researchers at the University of Iowa. Meanwhile, research in the UK shows that within 30 minutes of drinking a large cappuccino or expresso, the flow of blood to the brain is reduced by 10–20%. That's why you get that shaky, sweaty feeling after too many lattes.

23 Think About The Financial Benefits Of Quitting

Calculate how much you could save yourself if you broke a 20-a-day smoking habit, and then think about the things you could buy with the money. Think how much that would be over a lifetime!

24 Don't Be Fooled By Smoking Less

Although the more you smoke the greater the risk, just one or two cigarettes a day is more than enough to cause lung cancer (smoking-related lung cancer has risen by 70% in under 15 years). Plus, simply being in a smoky environment can damage your health. Passive smoking causes around 200 deaths a year.

25 Join The Quitter's Club

In the UK, 83% of people who give up smoking do it for health reasons. Worldwide, 10 million people kicked the habit last year!

chapter 4

The sex stuff

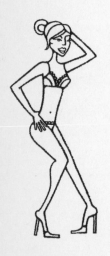

Do you ever stop to think about your sexual health? Or do you play the Let's-ignore-that-lump-until-it-goes-away game? If so, it's worth noting that sexual health is one area you just can't afford to be lazy about. You can get away with eating badly, drinking too much and not sleeping, but neglect your downstairs bits and you're heading for a future of trouble. So this chapter is a bit of a wake-up call to those who ditch their smear test reminders, can't be bothered to practise safer sex and ignore weird and not so wonderful symptoms – do yourself a favour and take note.

The good news

Even if you're so lazy you haven't yet signed up with a local doctor, your sexual health is still the easiest area of your wellbeing to deal with. Apart from the fact that you don't have to do much besides use condoms and keep your doctor's appointments, there are a multitude of free clinics just waiting to help you. And if you're unlucky enough to have bigger problems, a trip to your local (and hugely confidential) Genito-Urinary Medicine (GUM) clinic will soon sort you out. All of which means you've really got no excuse not to stay 100% sexually fit.

Why sex is good for your health

In Chinese medicine, sexual energy has long been associated with the basis of a person's emotional wellbeing. One study from the Institute of Human Sexuality found that the risk of death amongst those with a high orgasmic frequency was half that of people who had sex less than once a month. The reason is simple – sex is energetic and encourages the release of a number of feel-good chemicals in the body. An active sex life could be your way of getting fit, warding off illnesses, boosting your state of health, and erasing stress.

Here's what having sex twice a week can do:

Give you a healthy heart

Sex increases the maximum heart rate to about 120 beats a minute – that's the same as a fast walk/jog, which means you'll be unclogging arteries, lowering your risk of diabetes and lengthening your life. Having sex at this level three times a week for at least 20 minutes will reduce your risk of coronary heart disease by 50%. It will also lower your risk of ovarian, cervical and bowel cancer, and reduce your risk of Type II diabetes which affects 1.3 million people in the UK. Type II diabetes is triggered by weight and your diet as you get older.

Boost your immunity

New studies show that regular lovemaking boosts the production of antibodies in the body – your defence against disease. These germ-busting chemicals help you to fight off illnesses and stay cold-free. Sex, and orgasms in particular, means you are less likely to get colds, flu and stomach complaints.

Slow down the ageing process

Research by Italian scientists at the University of Rome has found that regular physical contact, from kissing to sex, is as important to longevity as exercise. Apparently, human contact is a powerful weapon against ageing because it releases the body's natural painkillers – endorphins – which increase the body's staying power.

Boost your libido

Both men and women who have sex regularly when they are young retain the physical capacity to do so when they are older. Studies show that if you don't give your libido regular exercise (whether this is through sex, masturbation or fantasy), you'll lose the urge totally as you get older.

Stop period pain

Weekly sex equals a more regular menstrual cycle, higher oestrogen levels and less PMS. Orgasm can also put a halt to period pain and painful cramps, and any vaginal or clitoral stimulation will produce a pain-blocking effect in the body.

The disappearing libido

We're all up for it all the time, right? Sadly not. Going off sex is as common as going off your food. If having sex seems like a huge effort not worth making, it pays to look behind the scenes.

Problem One: Your hormones are playing up

Progesterone is famous for lowering the sex drive, so if your libido has disappeared, see if you can trace it back to a time you started a new type of contraceptive, or another kind of medication such as an antidepressant (also renowned for lowering the libido). Then see your GP, because while certain contraceptive pills can affect your drive, there are over 30 different types of pill to choose from – meaning you'll find the brand that's right for you.

Problem Two: You're too tired

Living in the fast lane might be fun, but something's got to give eventually and it's likely to be your sex life. On average most people in their late 20s and early 30s (in the Western world) work an average of nearly 45 hours per week, and that's before you add in overtime and weekend working. If you play as hard as you work, you're going to find it difficult to heat up the sheets at night. This kind of fatigue interferes in a big way with your sex life because when the body is under stress, the part of your nervous system that deals with essential life-saving functions, like breathing, takes over and shuts down the less essential functions, like sexual pleasure.

"going off sex is as common as going off your food."

The answer is simple – give yourself more time. Find relaxation techniques that work for you: a long bath, calming music, TV, etc. Just 40 minutes of this twice a day will help re-energise your sex drive.

Problem Three: You're depressed

Depression affects one in five women in the UK. Key features include: lack of energy, despondency, loss of appetite and a loss of sexual desire. Depression is an illness and it needs to be treated by a doctor and/or counsellor. Your GP should be your first step as s/he can determine whether there is a physical reason for why you feel down. A counsellor can also help by treating you for the psychological aspects of your depression.

Problem Four: Sex is painful

Sometimes sex is painful because of a particular position or rhythm, e.g. deep thrusting; sometimes sex can hurt because you're not sufficiently lubricated, and sometimes there is an underlying medical reason for why intercourse is painful. If sex hurts, you first need to identify where the pain is.

- If it's inside the vaginal area, it could be lack of lubrication, a yeast infection, or a sexually transmitted infection (STI) such as trichomoniasis or vaginismus (spasms in the vaginal wall)
- If it's in the outer genital area, it could be a sexual infection, such as herpes or warts
- If it's deep in the pelvis, it could be the STI chlamydia (a dull ache), a bladder infection (a dull ache and frequent, painful urination), or endometriosis (constant pain that's worse during a period and sex)

If any of this sounds familiar go to the Genito-Urinary Medicine clinic (GUM) at your local hospital and get checked out.

Sexually transmitted infections (STIs)

You knew this bit was coming. Hopefully, you won't ever contract a sexually transmitted infection, but it pays to stay informed just in case.

Sexual danger signals

STI's don't always-present symptoms, but warning signs to watch out for are:

- The feeling you're peeing razor blades
- Lumps and bumps
- Blisters – small or large
- Discharges – watery, or lumpy
- Irritation – anywhere in the genital region
- Cauliflower-like swellings in the genital region
- Strange Smells – especially if it's fishy rashes around the genital area (not just the vagina, but the bottom and upper thighs)
- Pain during sex – contrary to popular belief this is not normal

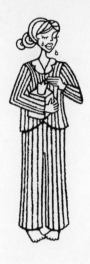

Why it happens

The Science Bit: Unfortunately, the female reproductive tract is an ideal environment for harbouring sexually transmitted infections. Not only is it warm and moist, the actual biology of the female genital tract positively lends itself to infection. The female urethra is shorter than the male (4 cm (1.5 in) long, compared to 20 cm (7.5 in)) which means the female urethral opening, vaginal opening and anal opening are all close together allowing bacteria easy access. This means we also suffer more serious consequences of STIs than men, because the infections travel further into our bodies. So if you are in your mid to late 20s, having unprotected sex at least three times a week you will not only triple your chance of an STI, but the likelihood of you getting pregnant in any one month will be over 30%.

What you can catch today

1. Genital warts

Also known as human papillmavirus (HPV), this is the disease you are most likely to catch if you have unprotected sex. The latest UK government statistics show that genital warts represented almost a quarter of all cases of STIs reported last year. You need to be especially wary of genital warts because visible warts are highly infectious and can be passed on not only through penetrative sex but also genital-to-genital contact. Warts can also be found outside the condom area on the scrotum, thighs, buttocks and/or anus, so wearing a condom won't necessarily help. Plus, some people who carry the wart virus may never develop any visible warts themselves, but they can still infect a sexual partner with the virus who might then, in turn, develop warts. If you notice something, seek help immediately. There is no cure yet for the actual infection, but the warts themselves can be treated effectively. For an HPV DNA text and treatment, go to your nearest GUM clinic.

Help Yourself By:

- Limiting your sexual partners

2. HIV and AIDS

According to a new MORI poll, 1 in 14 UK adults indulge in unprotected sex and 51% of UK women do not think about using condoms before starting a new sexual relationship. Not wise, considering the latest statistics show HIV infection is on the increase, especially amongst young heterosexuals. It might not be as prevalent as genital warts, but beware of what you can catch on your holidays. In certain countries, such as Italy, Spain and France, HIV rates are much higher than in the UK and in some African countries, like Kenya, as many as 1 in 4 are HIV positive. For a confidential HIV test, go to your nearest GUM clinic.

Help Yourself By:

- Practising safer sex
- Limiting your sexual partners

3. Chlamydia

Chlamydia trachomatis is the most common sexually transmitted bacterium in the UK. The latest government figures from the UK Public Health Laboratory show that cases of chlamydia amongst women have soared by almost 57% – 11,126 of these cases were found in women aged 20–34 (and 10,563 in men aged 20–34). In 80% of cases the sufferer shows no symptoms. Don't be tempted to ignore the threat of chlamydia as it has very serious long-term consequences. Left untreated, it can lead to pelvic inflammatory disease (PID), problems with fertility, heavier periods and pain during sex. If you've had unprotected sex in the past and are worried you may be infected, go to your nearest GUM clinic for a simple chlamydia test. If chlamydia is diagnosed, all you need is a single dose of antibiotics to clear it up.

Help Yourself By:

- Having protected sex.

4. A bacterial or urinary tract infection

Bacterial infections are not sexually transmitted (but can be passed on through sex). They include the very common infections, cystitis and thrush (see below), bladder infections, and bacterial vaginosis. Many of these infections can be treated over the counter, but it's wise not to self-diagnose. It's easy to assume a discharge is something you know, such as thrush, but beware – it could actually be one of the most common sexually transmitted vaginal infections, trichomoniasis. If you suspect you may be infected with anything, go to your nearest GUM clinic for a diagnosis.

Cystitis can be triggered by a number of things, such as sex, not drinking enough water and tight non-cotton underwear, which creates the perfect environment for bacteria. Symptoms include a burning pain when peeing, needing to pee a lot, blood in your pee, and back pain or a temperature. Sometimes you'll find you need to pee and can't.

Help Yourself By:
- Drinking a pint of water every 20 minutes for 3 hours during an attack. This will flush out your system
- Going to the toilet before and after sex. This will help flush out bacteria
- Avoiding caffeine and alcohol during an attack
- Avoiding sex until it's over
- Avoiding bath oils and bubble baths
- Drinking a few glasses of cranberry juice. It contains hippuric acid, which prevents bacteria from clinging to the lining of the urinary tract

Thrush is a fungal infection caused by Candida albicans. This fungus lives naturally in the stomach, but can multiply out of control if the natural flora of the stomach is upset by not eating properly, antibiotics or any kind of distress. It also develops quickly in hot climates and can be made worse by tight clothing, which provides an overheated environment where candida can grow. Symptoms include a lumpy white discharge (no smell), vaginal irritation and pain when peeing.

Help Yourself By:

- Having a salt-water bath to ease the itching
- Avoiding perfumed soaps and bubble baths
- Not having sex until it's cleared up, as you can infect your partner and he can re-infect you
- Seeing your doctor (or chemist if you know what it is) for anti-fungal pessaries, creams or tablets

tips

Help relieve cystitis by drinking a few glasses of cranberry juice. It contains hippuric acid, which prevents bacteria from clinging to the lining of the urinary tract.

5. Genital herpes

Genital herpes, like genital warts, has no cure. Herpes is caused by the herpes simplex II virus and is highly contagious. It can be transmitted through oral sex from a blister on the mouth to the genitals, from active blisters on the genital region and from people who have no apparent symptoms but carry the virus in their genital region. You need to see your doctor immediately if you feel numb or sensitive in the genital region, or if painful blisters or sores appear. While there is no cure, anti-viral treatments are effective in limiting the blisters.

Help Yourself By:

- Being vigilant if you're having sex with someone new

6. Gonorrhoea and syphilis

They may sound like diseases of old, but gonorrhoea and syphilis have not disappeared. In fact, according to the latest figures, 5,526 men aged 20–34 and 2,165 women in the same age group were diagnosed with gonorrhoea in 1996/97. This represents a 30% increase in cases from the year before. And while only 39 men and 14 women were diagnosed with syphilis, this is also a rise of 26%.

The big problem with gonorrhoea is that five out of every six women infected have no symptoms. Penicillin is the main treatment for both gonorrhoea and syphilis.

Help Yourself By:

- Having protected sex

Boost your chances of good sex

Eat properly

There's a lot to be said for aphrodisiacs. This doesn't mean you should stuff your face with oysters and asparagus every day, but there's no denying that the diet has a powerful effect on your sex drive. Eat foods high in sugar and saturated fat, washed down with caffeine and alcohol, and the chances are you'll only be up for it once a week (if you're lucky). To keep your hormones balanced, improve your energy in bed and keep your libido strong:

> *"diet has a powerful effect on your sex drive."*

- Keep to a relatively low fat diet
- Eat oily fish such as tuna, salmon and sardines at least twice a week
- Limit takeaway and processed foods to twice a week
- Reduce the salt in your food

Have a regular cervical smear

National screening for cervical cancer was only introduced in the UK in 1988, but now 4 million women are tested each year. The screening system is so efficient that every three years or so a note should come through your door telling you to make an appointment at your GP's. Neglect this at your peril, and remember that nowhere else in the world would you get this kind of health check for free and with a regular reminder from your doctor. Although horror stories about mistakes abound, the vast bulk of these smears are correctly interpreted, and the majority of women will be given the all clear.

The cervix is basically a very weak area of the female body, and during sex it's a meeting point for two different types of cell. This interaction can lead the cells of the cervix to change and become pre-cancerous (see below), which is why you need regular smears.

Lazy Tips For A Successful Smear:
- Relax and remind yourself this is not a cancer test but a test to pick up abnormal changes in the cervix. If there are

changes present, it's vital they're identified, because cervical cancer is associated with certain viruses that change the appearance of cervical cells. If changes can be detected at a very early stage, cancer can be avoided altogether. However, 92% of women tested get given the all clear

- Okay so they're uncomfortable, but they're not so bad that they're worth avoiding. To help yourself have a less painful test ask the nurse/doctor to warm the speculum before it's inserted. Nerves make many women tense up before the speculum is inserted, making it more uncomfortable and difficult to adjust. One way to make insertion easier is to concentrate on dropping your tailbone
- Avoid sex the night before you go for your appointment because semen makes the smear results unreliable
- Avoid going for your smear when you have a period because blood will also make the results unreliable

Take note of your periods

You can have an erratic menstrual cycle for a number of reasons: stress, weight problems, travel, even a change of job. But it pays not to be complacent. Any change, whether it is in the type of pain you're having, cycle length or consistency, could be a sign that you need to get your gynaecological health checked out.

1. Painful periods

Not all period pain is alike – cramps are divided medically into primary and secondary 'dysmenorrhoea':

tips

Take note of your periods. Any change, whether it is in the type of pain you're having, cycle length or consistency, could be a sign that you need to get your gynae-cological health checked out.

Primary dysmenorrhoea is caused by the release of the hormone prostaglandin in the uterus. This hormone helps propel the womb lining out of your body during your period, and works in spasms, hence the cramps. In 7% of women, too much prostaglandin is released and the cramps are so unbearable that sufferers cannot function at all on these days. Relief is found in the form of ibuprofen, and mefenamic acid (prescription only).

Secondary dysmenorrhoea is pain that lasts longer, has a higher than normal intensity and is caused, not by hormones, but by conditions such as uterine fibroids, a pelvic infection, or endo-metriosis – a migration of the uterine lining into other parts of your reproductive tract (see below). Killer cramps around your period and during sex may also indicate endometriosis.

Help Yourself By:

- Noting how your period pain has changed and when the pain occurs during the month. This information will help your doctor with diagnosis and treatment

2. Period blood

The blood expelled during your period should be a fairly normal red colour. Dark or old-looking blood before or at the end of a period can indicate a problem such as endometriosis. This is the second most common gynaecological problem in the UK, and affects over 2 million women. Around 30% of the women who have it will become infertile if they do not get treatment.

Endometriosis occurs when cells that are normally found in the lining of the uterus are deposited in other areas of the pelvic region, leading to pelvic pain and the formation of scar tissue in the pelvic region, and a loss of dark or old-looking blood during your period. Diagnosis can only be carried out with a laparoscopy. This is a minor operation in which a microscopic telescope (a laparoscope) is inserted into the pelvis via a small cut near the navel. It allows the doctor to see the pelvic organs clearly and diagnose the condition; it is then treated with a mixture of drugs and microsurgery.

3. Frequency

If your period cycle has always been regular and suddenly starts to come every two weeks, or less than once every five weeks (42 days), you may have a different problem.

Irregular periods, and erratic vaginal bleeding in particular, should always be taken very seriously. Either could be the result of polyps (small outgrowths from the endometrial or cervix cells) or another fertility-busting condition called polycystic ovarian syndrome (PCOS). Both polyps and PCOS could wreck your pregnancy plans.

Help Yourself By:

- Seeing your GP and asking for a referral to a gynaecologist

Perform a regular breast exam

Breast cancer may be on the increase but, with early treatment, it can be beaten, which is why it's important to examine your breasts monthly to detect any changes or lumps. Do it at the same time every month, just after your

"know what's normal for you."

periods, when your breasts are less lumpy. Remember, some women have naturally lumpy breasts – so don't panic if you find something.

Look after your breasts

The NHS Breast Screening Programme has produced a four-point plan to help women check for normality. If you want to make sure you stay healthy, consider the following:

1. Know what's normal for you. Every breast is different in texture and lumpiness – so get to know how yours feel. More importantly check at the same time every month.
2. Feel your breast area regularly. Moving in a circular motion, cover the whole breast, starting from deep in the armpit, then over the top of the breast tissue, centrally and underneath it, finally circling around and over the nipple. It is also important that you feel around the collarbone and into the armpit for any swellings.
3. Look for:
   - Changes to the appearance of your breast such as puckering and dimpling
   - Feelings of breast discomfort
   - Lumps. Don't expect these to be large. In 51% of cancer cases, lumps are less than 3 cm (1.25 in) across
   - Nipple discharges and changes in the nipple position
4. See your GP without delay if you are at all worried.

Look after your fertility

Okay, so a baby might be the last thing on your mind – but some time in the future you may change your mind. It's therefore worth noting that 1 out of 20 women younger than 30 have to 'work at' conceiving for more than a year. While infertility treatment is often successful, experts now believe you can protect your future fertility by gaining better overall health before you even think of getting pregnant. It means that when you're ready, your fertilisation rate will be higher and your womb lining healthier.

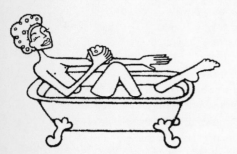

Good nutritional health improves the chances of conception because the food we eat has a direct impact on every part of our body. A healthy diet is vital if you want to conceive and give birth to a healthy baby.

Up Your Chances Of Conception By:

- Eating a wide range of fruit and vegetables
- Including more oily fish in your diet, such as sardines, tuna and mackerel. They are an essential source of Omega 3 and 6 fatty acids, which are vital for hormonal balance
- Adding soya to your diet in the form of tofu or soya milk. Soya is classed as a phyto-oestrogen, which means it contains substances that act like hormones. It has been shown to balance the sex hormones and prevent heavy or long periods

- Eating less meat, because the saturated fat in animal products stimulates oestrogen production, which reduces your chance of conceiving
- Upping your zinc levels. Zinc is essential for maintaining the healthy creation of cells. The recommended daily dose is 15 mg and the best natural sources are wholemeal bread, cheese, poultry, tuna, eggs and beans
- Giving up smoking. Tobacco and nicotine can affect fertility levels by as much as 50%
- Cutting back on drink. Meanwhile, alcohol has been shown to poison sperm and damage ovum before conception
- Learning to relax. Studies have shown that stress can affect a woman's ability to conceive and, in extreme cases, can stop her ovulating

Get your other half checked out

Guys are notoriously bad at going to the doctor's for their general health, never mind their sexual health. Which is why direct tactics should be taken with them (i.e. don't beat about the bush!).

- Always use a condom – no matter how nice he looks if he doesn't know what's going on down below, you certainly won't
- Men rarely present symptoms of STIs. If you've found yourself with something nasty, get him checked out too and don't have sex until you are both infection-free (or you'll re-infect each other)

- Men can also get thrush so the same advice applies – avoid sex until you're both clear or you'll just keep re-infecting each other
- Make him aware of testicular cancer – the commonest form of cancer in men aged 20–40. The good news is that 95% of those affected can be cured if the cancer is caught early. Most testicular cancer tumours (80%) first appear as swellings in the balls, so he should examine himself regularly and see a doctor for an ultrasound if he finds anything

Take care with contraception

What's your excuse for not using contraception – too lazy to unwrap it, too busy to go to your doctor's? It makes you sick/tired/sore/fed up? Whatever your gripe, it's worth remembering that contraception could save your life.

Popular Pill Myths:

- It makes you put on weight
- It's bad for your health
- It causes mood swings
- It decreases your fertility
- It turns you off sex

There are 33 brands of contraceptive pill currently available and 23 different types, so even if one pill gives you problems, the chances are you'll find one that won't. For instance, if you're prone to acne, the progestogen in certain pills may make the condition worse. Minulet, Femodene and Brevinor all contain lower levels of pro-gestogen and are, therefore, less likely to cause acne. Weight gain is a big pill fear for many women, but this was really only a problem with the higher dose pills given out in the '60s. Not only is the pill 99% effective as a contraception (the 1% being down to human error), recent evidence shows that, as well as giving you regular periods, it lowers your risk of breast cancer, ovarian cancer and endometrial cancer.

Popular Condom Myths:

- They make sex less enjoyable
- They are too small for well-endowed men
- They limit orgasm
- They split easily

Condoms are now thinner and stronger than they've ever been. They only tear when they are snagged by jewellery or sharp nails, and are ineffective only if you don't remove them properly. Latex condoms also weaken if you use them with Vaseline or any oil-based lubricant so beware of bath oils, moisturisers and hand cream. Water-based lubricants are best. Also, store condoms away from heat as this weakens them. As for size – condoms can stretch to way over a metre – need I say more?

Popular Emergency Contraception Myths:

- It's hard to get
- It's bad for you
- It doesn't work
- There's not enough time to get it
- You can only take it the morning after

tips

Boost your orgasm potential: For better orgasms, excercise your pelvic floor muscles (the ones you pee with). Clench and release 20 times a day and build up to 50.

There are two ways of preventing pregnancy after unprotected sex and both have to be started within 1–5 days, which is long enough for anyone to get to a chemist or doctor (though the sooner you sort it out the better the contraceptive will work).

1. Levonelle-2

This is a new and more effective form of the emergency contraceptive pill (generally known as the 'morning-after pill'). It has to be taken within 72 hours of unprotected sex. Unlike its predecessor, PC4 – the oestrogen and progestogen emergency pill – Levonelle-2 contains progestogen only and comes in a two-pill form (rather than the old four-pill make up that PC4 came in). The old side effects of nausea and vomiting are practically non-existent, so you don't need to worry about it affecting your general health.

You can now buy Levonelle-2 over the counter at your local chemist. It's good news for the 170,000 UK women who end up having abortions each year, 90% percent of whom say they would have used emergency contraception had they been able to get it in time. Remember that the emergency pill stops conception occurring, and is not an abortion pill.

2. IUD

If you've waited beyond 72 hours but under five days, an IUD can be inserted by a doctor into the uterus to prevent the lining of the womb from thickening – therefore putting a halt to conception. This is an effective post-sex method and it's contraceptive value can last three years (or you can have it taken out again).

Go for a sexual health check up

Many GP surgeries now run Well Woman clinics, which will carry out smear and chlamydia testing. If you want something more in-depth, you can opt for a private Well Woman check at a Marie Stopes clinic (see Resources) for £100, which will include an HPV test. However, to get the 100% all clear, by far your best bet is a check at your nearest GUM clinic, where you can be tested and treated for all STIs.

If the thought of going to a sexual health clinic (GUM) makes you feel positively sick, let me reassure you that you have nothing to worry about. This is about the most confidential place you're ever likely to visit. For starters, even though these clinics are usually situated in a hospital, the records held here never leave the clinic. They are not placed with your normal hospital records or sent to your GP. No one will ever known you've been.

25 *ways* to a better sex life

1 Have Sex At Least Once A Week
Research shows that having sex at least once a week helps keep illness and depression away. It seems that genital stimulation makes for a stronger immune system, relieves headaches and combats the aches and pains of everyday life.

2 Don't Freak About No-shows
Contrary to popular belief, erections are not under a guy's voluntary control, and this is why the commonest causes of no-shows are tiredness and stress. Statistics show that one man in seven (aged 16 and above) has this type of erection problem at least four times a year.

3 Minimise Distractions During Sex
Watching television in bed has recently been voted the biggest libido killer. The flicker of the TV screen apparently hypnotises you into wanting sleep, desensitises you to sex and kills off your sex drive for the night. So if you want better sex, switch off and turn over.

4 Boost Your Orgasm Potential
For better orgasms, exercise your pelvic floor muscles. Also known as the PC (pubococcygeus) muscles, these are the ones you use to pee with. All you need to do is isolate the muscle. Do this by stopping your pee mid-flow, holding for five and then releasing. Once you've got the feel of them, clench and release 20 times a day (at your desk, on the bus, watching TV), and build up to 50.

5 Find Your G-spot
The elusive g-spot needn't be so elusive if you know exactly what to look for. The trick is to only search for it during sex, as this is when it becomes raised. Insert a finger into the vagina, move upwards about 5 cm and feel the front of the vaginal wall. Feel for a small textured bump and, lo and behold, that's your g-spot.

6 Master Your Body's Erogenous Zones

Erogenous zones – the body's sex sensors – are found all over the body and not just in the genital region. Caressed properly, these areas can give you the right kind of shudder during foreplay, sex and even after sex.

7 Have Regular Health Screenings

Nothing can kill your sex life faster than pelvic pain, pre-period pain and itchy, mysterious discharges. If you have any symptoms you are worried about (even a strange smell), get checked out by your doctor, even if you're 100% positive it's not an STI.

8 Re-assess Your Contraception

We all know condoms are the only way to protect against STIs and HIV, but with new contraceptive methods coming on the market all the time it pays to stay informed. Even if you've previously tried a method with little luck, it's worth going back to see what's new.

9 Change the Missionary Position

Improve on the classic man-on-top, woman-on-bottom position by keeping your legs straight and close together as he lies between your thighs.

10 Forget The Sex Statistics

Sex therapists say that if you want a better sex life, start by ignoring sex statistics about how often other people have sex. It only leads to feelings of sexual insecurity and worthlessness, which in turn leads to a decline in your sex life.

11 Change Positions

Eighty per cent of people use the missionary as their number one sex position. To get more out of sex, get on top of things – literally.

12 Bring A Banana To Bed

But not for the reason you're thinking. Bananas are a rich source of vitamin B and eating them therefore helps enhance both sex and orgasm by promoting the flow of blood to your sex organs.

13 Don't Kiss Each Other If You Have A Cold Sore

Cold sores on the mouth are a form of

herpes. They are a different strain from genital herpes, but if you dive south when you have one on your lip, you could end up giving your partner genital herpes as the virus can mutate on contact.

14 Be Selective About Food During Sex

Your vagina is not like your mouth, and even though they do it in the films, you shouldn't just put whatever you want in there and hope for the best.

15 Use A Condom During Your Period

Sex when you have your period is a matter of personal preference. If you're going for it, use condoms because the cervix is more open at this time and therefore more susceptible to infection.

16 Talk About Your Fantasies

It will turn you both on quicker than foreplay. If you're stuck for something to say, ask him to go first.

17 Don't Gossip About Your Sex Life

Surprisingly, chatting with your friends about what goes on in the bedroom can have a detrimental effect on your sex life. Firstly, most men consider a sex revelation told in jest to be a bit of a major betrayal. Secondly, compare and contrast stories have been shown to be a major self-esteem deflator.

18 Don't Imagine Size Doesn't Matter

Size does matter but not in the way guys think. A well-endowed partner thrusting too deeply or too quickly could mark the end of your sexual relationship and give you post-sex soreness. The key here is to go slow and use lots of lubrication. If the reverse is true, and your partner is on the small side, try positions that give deeper penetration, such as sex from behind.

19 Forget Simultaneous Orgasms

They always manage it in films – but that's because they're faking it (yes, even in porn films). The real chance of the two of you screaming the house down together is low, and trying too hard to achieve this will make your chances of orgasm non-existent, never mind simultaneous.

20 Talk Yourself Into Better Sex

It's estimated that 90% of people who have bad sex lives have them because they find talking about sex too embarrassing. Worried your partner can't handle the criticism? You might be surprised at his reaction. In a recent sex survey, 95% of men said they wished their girlfriends talked more about what they liked and disliked in bed.

21 Exercise Three Times A Week

Not just for better wellbeing, but because it improves your sex drive, your orgasm potential and your sexual staying power.

22 Have Sex In The Morning

There's a definite daily rhythm to the male sex hormone testosterone. Normally, levels are higher in the morning (as you can probably tell), lower in the late afternoon (when he starts to get tired), and very low at night (when he needs to sleep).

23 Know Your Monthly Hormonal Highs

It will help you to get the best out of your sex life. Days 7–14 in a regular cycle are the high point of the sexual month.

24 It will give you an instant face lift

Remind yourself that having sex three times a week can take 7 –12 years off your looks. But casual sex, because it's loaded with stress, will have the opposite effect.

25 Masturbate More

Masturbation is the perfect cure for a lot of life's problems, such as stress and anxiety. It's especially good if you have problems reaching orgasm or if your boyfriend is a premature ejaculator. Sex educators say it's the perfect tool to help you discover what works for you in bed, and what doesn't. If you think no one else does it, think again – 90% of people say they masturbate at least once a week.

chapter 5
Moody blues

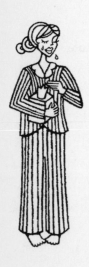

Mood swings, depression and the blues, even the non-lazy suffer from these feelings – but living it up, not getting enough shut-eye and ignoring what you put into your body can all contribute to the severity of your down times. So if you're feeling blue and don't know why, this chapter can help – and you won't have to put in hours of therapy, self-analysis and/or reach for those magic happy pills.

The truth behind your Dr Jekyll and Mr Hyde persona

Pre-menstrual syndrome (PMS)

The symptoms of PMS usually occur 5–10 days before your period, sometimes earlier. Symptoms include:

- Tearfulness
- Food cravings
- Mood swings
- Depression
- Bloating
- Painful breasts
- Irritability
- Weight gain
- Headaches
- Sleep and concentration problems
- Anger

Although PMS can happen at any age, it's extremely common between the ages of 25 and 40, and you're twice as likely to suffer from it if your mother did. According to the latest statistics, PMS affects up to 80% of women before they reach the menopause and, while the severity and range of symptoms (there are 150 recognised ones) might vary from one period to another, the sufferer can always identify at least five symptoms each month.

There are many theories about what causes PMS. The only thing that's known for sure is that it can be triggered by fluctuating levels of hormones prior to your period – too much oestrogen and too little progesterone. As for the emotional aspects, PMS tends to bring on the same problems you can usually deal with or push away in everyday non-PMS life. Which is why some people get down about their relationships, others about money and some about their bodies.

The good news is that there are some easy ways to get rid of PMS, and they really do work!

For bloating . . . start by trying not to freak out – our bodies store water so that they don't get dehydrated before a period arrives. To help reduce this water retention, cut your levels of salt, caffeine and alcohol prior to your period.

For weight gain . . . again, don't worry – it's due to excess fluid that will be expelled with your period. Plus, it's unlikely you'll put on any weight even if you're scoffing madly because the body needs this extra energy to get you through your period (see below).

For appetite changes . . . don't starve yourself. Your body needs an extra 500 calories a day prior to your period.

For mild to moderate blues . . . exercise and dietary supplements such as vitamin B6, calcium and magnesium can help make you feel better. However, don't be impatient – they won't work instantaneously. Try taking them for three months to see good results.

For moderate blues and PMS . . . the contraceptive pill is often prescribed and works for many women.

For severe symptoms and PMS . . . Prozac has been shown in a number of studies to be successful because it raises levels of serotonin in the brain (found to be low in PMS sufferers), and helps you to regain control of your life.

For irritability and tension . . . do some exercise. Not only will this release feel-good endorphins into your bloodstream and make you feel better, it will also help with abdominal cramps and joint aches.

"have a good cry — studies show it's good for you."

For tearfulness . . . have a good cry – studies show it's good for you.

For severe depression . . . seek the help of a counsellor, even if it only hits you in the second half of your menstrual cycle.

For breast tenderness . . . wear a roomier bra – it will help more than you could ever imagine.

For chocolate cravings . . . give in – even if it doesn't actually help, it tastes good.

For PMS in general . . . take a calcium supplement. Several studies show it can reduce PMS symptoms by as much as 50%.

Your hormones

You go from feeling very happy and carefree to feeling tired and blue. Two female sex hormones, oestrogen and progesterone, rule us all. Oestrogen is the sultry sex kitten of hormones – sexy, vivacious, and desperate for attention. Progesterone is her moody, stroppy sister – eager to smother those flames of passion and spoil all your fun. If you're feeling weirdly sad, depressed, bloated, sentimental, mad, or just plain bored all in the space of one day, it's likely that one of these hormones is to blame.

To help you cope, take a look at your hormonal month:

Days 1–7. (taken from the day your period starts). You're likely to be relaxed, happy and calm. This is all down to the release of a hormone from the brain's pituitary gland called FSH (follicle stimulating hormone). FSH stimulates your ovaries, which means your stress levels will be at an all-time low and your concentration levels fantastic.

Days 7–14. You're heading towards the storm of ovulation. It's the highlight of your sexual month so you will feel at your most attractive and sexy.

Days 14–21. Initially, the release of what is known as 'luteinizing' hormone in the brain will trigger ovulation and boost your libido to an all-time high. However, once ovulation has occurred (this process takes about two days) your oestrogen levels will drop and progesterone will start to rise, killing your sex drive and bringing on the PMS blues.

Days 21—28. The PMS days – prepare yourself, because your two favourite sex hormones have dropped out of sight. Your concentration levels are low as your body's energies have been processed into other areas of your body. The better news is that testosterone (the male sex hormone) gets a small look in (we all have small amounts of this naturally present in our bodies) and, mixed with decreasing levels of oestrogen, this will give you a sudden sexual surge, which means you'll be incredibly orgasm-friendly!

Anaemia

Anaemia is a condition which results from the body not being able to produce enough haemoglobin (a protein that carries oxygen to the red blood cells and to the tissues in the body). When this happens, a person is left with no energy and feels drained, depressed and irritable. Other symptoms are fatigue, dizziness, fainting spells, apathy, irritability, a decreased ability to concentrate and intolerance to the cold. Nearly 20% of women are at risk from becoming anaemic, for the following reasons:

- Not enough iron in their diets (found in red meat, spinach and green leafy vegetables)
- Excessive dieting

- Heavy bleeding during a period
- Too much alcohol

Your doctor is the best person to diagnose anaemia, simply because fatigue and depression can often mask other illnesses (so never self-diagnose and start taking iron supplements off your own bat). Anaemia is diagnosed with a blood test, which will reveal your body's iron levels. If you are low in iron, your doctor is likely to recommend iron supplements and an iron-rich diet.

Help Yourself By:

- Upping the iron in your diet. Women need 15 mg of iron a day. You can make your diet iron-rich by eating meat, fish, dried apricots, sardines, chicken, tofu, spinach and breakfast cereals

Low blood sugar

Eating foods that cause sugar levels in the body to drop or rise too quickly causes low blood sugar (see Chapter 1), resulting in mood fluctuation. The foods to blame are, of course, all your favourites: chocolate, refined carbohydrates, coffee, processed foods and sugary desserts. However, you'll be comforted to know that true hypoglycaemia (low blood sugar) affects less than 2% of the population.

Help Yourself By:

- Getting an accurate diagnosis of low blood sugar, which can be done with a simple blood-sugar test at your GP's
- Eating small meals every three hours

tips

When you need a snack, eat a banana as it will release its sugar in small doses, helping your blood sugar levels to stabilise.

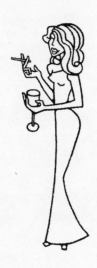

- Eating foods like bananas when you need a snack – unlike chocolate, which releases sugar in one big explosion because it is refined sugar, a banana will release sugar into your body in small doses, helping your blood sugar levels to stabilise
- Remember that if you fill up on a lot of sugar-laden food, the chances are you are not getting enough essential nutrients. Being deficient in calcium, magnesium and B vitamins (especially B6) can all cause depression, because these nutrients all manufacture hormones and neurotransmitters (emotional messages from the brain to the rest of the body)

Seasonal affective disorder (SAD)

It is estimated that as many as 10% of the general population suffer from winter depression, otherwise known as Seasonal Affective Disorder (SAD). Researchers believe that this type of depression is caused by the lack of natural daylight at this time of year, because light has a biological effect on the brain's hormones, particularly serotonin and dopamine which control the brain's mood chemicals. Light deprivation affects the production of these chemicals, bringing on depression, low energy, an increased need for sleep, an increased appetite for comforting foods, and reduced concentration.

Help Yourself By:

- Spending more time outside in natural light, which can relieve milder symptoms

- Trying something known as light therapy, or phototherapy, which involves exposure to bright, artificial light. As little as 30 minutes per day spent sitting under this kind of light is said to bring about an improvement in 60–80% of SAD sufferers. Lightboxes cost from £200 and are not available on the NHS (see Resources for details of SAD association)
- Going to see your doctor, who can offer you various treatments for winter depression such as counselling or antidepressant medications

Irritable bowel syndrome (IBS)

Bloating, cramp-like stomach pain, tiredness, feeling low – do these sound all too familiar? If so, you may well be suffering from IBS. This disorder of the intestines is now such a common condition that as much as a quarter of the population is suffering with it. What's more, most sufferers are aged between 20 and 40, and two out of three are female.

IBS is essentially a disturbance of the intestinal tract (colon). Under normal conditions, the intestinal tract pushes waste along in ordered contractions towards the rectum. But with IBS these contractions are uncoordinated, causing painful cramps, bloating, gas, constipation and diarrhoea. Doctors don't know exactly what causes this condition, although it's believed that stress is a factor, along with a more sensitive than usual colon, which causes the muscles in the gut to go, automatically, into spasm.

Help Yourself By:

- Learning to control your stress levels. The link between IBS and stress is pretty clear so this should be your first step. Experts recommend that relaxing alone for 20 minutes a day, regular exercise (20 minutes, three times a week) and learning your own limitations can all help create a more stress-free life

- Keeping a food diary. Food intolerance can also bring on IBS – wheat and dairy products being the most frequent offenders. This is because the gut cannot break down foods it is intolerant to, leading to bloating, cramps and excessive gas. If you think this might be the problem, try eliminating these foods for two weeks, checking your body's response and then introducing them slowly back into your diet. The best way to do this is to keep a food diary, noting which foods seem to cause you most distress and at what times. You can then consult a dietician or your doctor, who can help you make changes accordingly

- Getting a prescription. While IBS cannot be cured, your doctor can prescribe you any of the following: antispasmodics – alevrine or mebeverine – which will relax the bowel and help calm spasms; peppermint capsules, to help prevent bloating and wind; anti-diarrhoeal tablets, to relieve loose bowel movements

- Eating smaller meals, more often. This will keep the gut from becoming overloaded. Keep meals low in fat and starch, and high in carbohydrates

- Taking regular exercise. Increasing the amount of exercise you take will help the bowel have more regular motions and relieve bloating

Candida

Candida is an imbalance of gut bacteria caused by the multiplication of a yeast naturally present in every man, woman and child. In a normal healthy person, the number of candida organisms is controlled within the body and causes no trouble whatsoever. However, when a person becomes unwell and/or under stress, the immune system is weakened and normal candida in the body multiplies. This huge yeast overload then blocks food digestion, causing food to ferment and bringing on a condition known as 'leaky gut'. When this occurs, toxins from the gut leak into the bloodstream, leading to a whole host of symptoms including depression, abdominal bloating, fatigue, wind, diarrhoea, constipation, skin problems and persistent thrush.

Help Yourself By:

- Getting expert help. Candida needs proper diagnosis with laboratory tests. If your GP won't do it (some doctors refuse to recognise candida as a condition), you need to go through an alternative practitioner, who will rely on a thorough health history and a physical examination to determine if you have this illness. If you do have candida, you will probably be given anti-yeast medication and put on the 'anti-candida' diet. This diet works on the principle that you can rid your body of candida by starving the yeast that lives on the sugars you eat. It therefore involves banning a huge amount of things you normally eat and drink, including all sugar, fruit and alcohol

Sleeping difficulties

If you're tired all the time, can't wake up or can't go to sleep, the chances are you're also feeling depressed, irritable and tense about life. Most of us underestimate how lack of sleep affects our moods and makes us feel miserable and tearful. The average person needs about eight hours. Regularly deprive yourself of sleep and you'll reduce your ability to make decisions, handle complex tasks and think rationally.

> "Most of us under-estimate how lack of sleep affects our moods"

Insomnia, on the other hand, is a condition where you can't sleep despite deep fatigue. It affects one in three of us at some point in our lives and as a woman you are 1.3 times more likely to suffer from it. Studies show it also leads to depression, lower immunity, a drop in concentration levels, and even a reduced IQ.

Are you getting enough sleep?

Do any of the following apply to you?
- You need an alarm to wake you up
- You fall asleep at 9 pm watching TV
- You still feel tired after eight hours sleep
- You fall asleep as soon as your head hits the pillow
- Some days you feel like you could sleep at your desk
- You can't wait for the moment you go to bed

If you can tick two or more of the above, you need more sleep!

Help Yourself By:

- Going to bed half an hour earlier
- Not watching TV in bed, as experts say this tricks your body into staying awake and hyped up
- Not eating anything that is difficult to digest in the two hours before you go to bed as this will keep you awake
- Working out if you're caffeine sensitive – if so, stop drinking tea and coffee after 4 pm
- Napping if you need to – a 10-minute nap after you finish work and before you go out will improve your mood because the body's energy levels dip naturally and need time to build up again
- Going to see your GP to discuss possible underlying problems. If your insomnia lasts for more than a week and you don't know why, it's time to see a doctor

Your diet

Depressed about your weight? Well, go on a very low fat diet, and you'll feel even worse. Diet-related depression occurs in women who have a low intake of polyunsaturated fats (as opposed to the saturated fats that are found in meat, butter and cheese). This is because Omega 3, an essential fatty acid, which is found in fish, protects against depression. Studies show that the fatty acid found in fish is essential for feeling good. Rates of depression have risen steadily over the decades as the proportion of fish eaten has declined in people's food intake. (For more detail on saturated and unsaturated fats, see Chapter 1.)

Help Yourself By:

- Eating more fatty fish – salmon, halibut, tuna and sardines. Or take a fish oil supplement
- Eating the right amount of carbohydrate (5–7 servings a day) because serotonin (an essential chemical that regulates mood) drops in the body if you don't

Snoring

Snoring of the floorboard-rattling kind is not a male prerogative. The ratio of men to women who snore is actually 4:1.

Snoring is bad news because it disrupts sleep without you knowing it, meaning you wake up grumpy and have no reason why. Plus, it's embarrassing. You can blame all the noise on the vibration of air passing over a loose soft palate, i.e. the bit that hangs down near your tonsils.

Help Yourself By:

- Keeping your body weight down. The more fat you have around your throat, the more your palate will be squashed and restricted when you're asleep
- Avoiding alcohol for up to four hours before you sleep – it reduces the tone in your throat muscles making you snore louder
- Not smoking – it inflames the lining of the nose, restricting breathing
- Not sleeping on your back – your tongue will roll back and obstruct your airway

Particularly loud snorers will suffer 'sleep apnoea syndrome'. Sufferers have extremely disrupted sleep and wake up many times during the night (often without realising it), choking or with shortness of breath, caused by the throat narrowing and little or no air getting through. If you are excessively tired during the day and irritable and restless at night, this could be the problem.

Allergies

Food-related allergies or intolerance are another reason why your mood may shift and leave you feeling low and lethargic. Allergies – which refer to any hypersensitive reaction to any substance – are on the increase in the UK.

The British Allergy Foundation say allergic disorders affect up to 40% of the UK population and are increasing by 5% each year.

Food intolerance is when your body can't tolerate a particular food, or part of the food. Symptoms then arise, including headaches, stomach cramps and low mood. Unlike an allergy, which causes a specific reaction in the body that can be observed, food intolerance does not show itself obviously, which makes it hard to test for (and is why some doctors won't accept it exists).

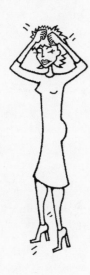

Help Yourself By:
Seeing your GP immediately if you get any of the following symptoms, and they become increasingly severe:

- An itchy rash – like nettle rash
- Faintness
- Swellings in the mouth
- Swelling in the throat
- Vomiting
- Cramping
- Diarrhoea
- A tingling feeling in the mouth and lips
- A sense of dread
- Disorientation
- Weakness and floppiness
- Asthmatic signs

Allergy testing is done via a skin prick test, or a blood test known as the Radio-Allergosorbent test. Testing indicates the degree of reactivity to a specific substance and so gives you guidance on the severity of your allergy. The British Allergy Foundation recommend the skin prick test because they say it is the most accurate. However, there are many other techniques used in alternative medicine for identifying allergies (most of which aren't recognised by traditional practitioners). For a list of reputable alternative practitioners, contact the British Institute for Allergy & Environmental Therapy (see Resources).

Diabetes

You feel cranky, fatigued and unusually blue. Signs of depression or PMS? Don't be so sure – undiagnosed diabetes will give you the same symptoms and a few more (increased thirst and a need urinate frequently). In the UK 2.3 million people currently suffer from diabetes and over a million of them don't realise they have it. Leave your symptoms unchecked and you are in danger of damaging your blood vessels, heart, kidneys and eyes. If detected early, diabetes can be controlled and damage to the body can be limited.

Help Yourself By:

- Having a test at your GP's. It's a simple blood or urine test (though the blood test is more accurate), and it's available free on the NHS

Depression

Of course, there is another, more common reason for feeling blue and it's called depression. Studies show it's likely to hit one in four of us in our lifetime, and the World Health Organization estimates that depression currently affects 340 million people worldwide. Worse still, there's no guaranteed way of avoiding it – being rich won't help, neither will being famous or beautiful, or in a good relationship!

Symptoms of depression

Depression is said to exist when you have had a low mood for more than two weeks and have at least three of the following symptoms:
- Feeling tired all the time
- Feelings of hopelessness
- Appetite changes
- Constant fear and anxiety
- Tearfulness
- Difficulty doing routine things
- Difficulty concentrating
- Feelings of self-blame and self-criticism
- Low confidence and self-esteem
- Sleep problems
- Persistent negative thoughts
- Persistent low moods
- Suicidal thoughts

"whatever the cause of depression, 80% of cases can be successfully treated."

The good news is that whatever the cause of your depression, 80% of cases can be successfully treated. Although it's important to realise there are no quick fixes, there are a variety of treatments available and your GP can help you find your way through the options.

1. Drug Therapy

You may be offered an antidepressant – a drug that can help alleviate depression. The most commonly prescribed antidepressant is currently Prozac, which has been used by more than 37 million people worldwide, and by 1 million people in the UK. Prozac is one of a new class of antidepressants known as selective serotonin re-uptake inhibitors (SSRIs). They work by increasing levels of the brain chemical serotonin (depressed people have been found to have low levels of this), which leads to improved mood.

However, like all medications, Prozac is not a wonder pill, and apart from the fact that it has side effects – including nausea, insomnia, dry mouth and, in some cases, a decreased libido – it isn't a permanent solution to depression. The aim with antidepressants is to take a course of medication for around six months, and recover to a point where you can seek other methods of coping, such as counselling.

2. Natural medicine

If you prefer the idea of something natural, it's worth noting that in a new clinical study, the so-called herbal equivalent to antidepressants – St John's wort – has been found to be ineffective in treating depression. Whatever you're considering, it's essential you see your GP before opting for complementary treatment. Some herbal and homeopathic treatments interact badly with conventional medicines, such as the contraceptive pill, other antidepressants and heart condition medication, so never be fooled by the notion that natural is safe.

The reason why herbal remedies aren't prescribed is because they aren't licensed. This means they have not been put through rigorous testing and procedures to establish their effectiveness, and most of their 'success' is anecdotal. This isn't to say that alternative treatments, such as acupuncture and reflexology, (see Chapter 8) don't work.

3. Therapy

Two recent US studies have shown that talking therapies can alleviate the symptoms of depression and last longer than anti-depressants. While there are hundreds of different types of therapy, all counselling approaches ultimately have the same goal: to help you feel better by bringing the stuff on the inside on to the outside.

In the UK you can receive free counselling on the NHS. See your GP – 60% of UK surgeries now have counsellors attached. However, financial constraints mean that waiting lists are long.

tips

Help motivate yourself with daily challenges that give you a sense of achievement.

The government has also limited the amount of time you can see a counsellor and you won't usually get more than six sessions. If you're willing to pay, your best option is go through the British Association of Counselling (BAC, see Resources) because counseling is not a regulated profession in the UK.

There are central bodies in most countries which can be contacted in order to find a councellor. Going through an organisation which regulates its membership, will ensure that you end up with someone who has gone through an ethical procedure, and has had proper training.

25 *ways* to boost your mood

1 Fake It
Your mood that is – smile, laugh, guffaw loudly and act silly for two minutes. Going through the motions is said to help trigger and harness happy thoughts that will boost your mood and make you feel better.

2 Take Some Vitamins
Vitamins B_6 and B_3 are essential for the production of serotonin. Zinc supports the balance of neurotransmitters in the brain and can also help alleviate low mood.

3 Declutter Your Life
Sounds bizarre, but sorting out your wardrobe, drawers and magazines, and throwing out all that accumulated rubbish will make you feel better. The stricter you are about it, the higher the benefit. Think of it as cathartic cleansing.

4 Make A List
Start your morning by writing down three things you want to accomplish by the end of the day. Studies show that people feel happier when they feel they have achieved something, no matter how small.

5 Beat PMS
If you want some natural relief from PMS, try agnus castus – a new study shows that taking this herbal supplement can improve PMS by up to 50% by balancing your hormones.

6 Pay Your Bills On Time
Studies on low mood show that leaving essential things undone and unfinished in your life (like bills) drains energy, causes anxiety and creates unnecessary tension.

7 Walk The Talk
Don't procrastinate, and don't say it if you don't mean to do it. You're just adding to your life's clutter.

8 Eat To Sleep

Still awake at 2 am? Get up and make yourself a turkey sandwich and wash it down with a glass of milk – the trytophan in them will help produce the essential sleep chemicals.

9 Live Near The Sea

Sea air is rich in tranquillising bromide ions and these mixed with the sound of water will generate feelings of overall wellbeing and help you formulate a regular sleeping pattern.

10 Take Kava Kava

If you can't sleep, feel anxious and worry needlessly all night, try taking the herbal supplement kava kava four hours before you go to bed. Studies show it will help you to relax and fall asleep more easily.

11 Don't Lie In At Weekends

Staying in bed at weekends or trying to catch up on late nights with long lie-ins just confuses your body's internal clock. It's light that resets your body's timer not more sleep. If you do lie in, help stop the crankiness by going out into the sunlight as soon as you get up.

12 Have A Good Laugh

Watch your favourite video. Laughter has the same invigorating effects as a quick run: it lowers the tension levels in your body, relaxes your muscles and releases much needed feel-good endorphins that will make you feel happier.

13 Don't Whinge

One way to keep yourself down is to whinge constantly about your problems. While talking about them is good if you're trying to find a solution, being a drama queen about an incident/event just makes you brood on negative feelings and relive them over and over.

14 Don't Aim For Perfection

Perfection is impossible in normal everyday life, so trying to meet impossibly high standards is a waste of time. Instead, aim to be realistic and go with the flow – it will make you much happier.

15 Have More Fun

Work less, worry less and go out and use your free time just for fun – it will make you feel less depressed, more connected to others and will improve your wellbeing generally.

16 Accept The Things You Cannot Change

For instance, your height, your colouring, the fact you haven't won the lottery and are not an Oscar-winning actress. It will make you feel less blue and more positive about your future.

17 Learn To Say No

This is about not taking on more than you can handle. Say yes to everything and you'll be overwhelmed, put upon and depressed about the fact that everyone always leans on you.

18 Let Go Of The Past

Including mistakes, dodgy boyfriends, stupid things you've done – learn from it and move on, instead of reminding yourself about it and letting it drag you down.

19 Suspend Judgement

Studies show that being judgemental about other people and their actions is a sign you are hyper self-critical. For an easier life, don't view yourself as good or bad, give yourself a break and admit you're human.

20 Throw Something

Indulge in some crockery throwing – it's good for your heart and mind. Apparently, a third of high blood pressure sufferers have repressed anger. The solution, say the experts, is better out than in!

21 Do Something You Enjoy

Research from the Science of Enjoyment found that indulging in anything you enjoy, be it shopping or loafing, boosts your immune system, relieves emotional tension and raises serotonin levels in the brain.

22 Ask More Questions

Sounds weird but higher

curiosity levels mean you adapt better to change, stress and challenges. It also helps keep your mind on external issues and not on internal 'me, me, me' issues.

23 Stand Up

Feeling tired and blue? Don't lie down as this will just make you feel worse. Standing up means you'll be more alert, be able to think faster, problem solve and remain active – all of which will stimulate the brain and make you feel better in general.

24 Do All Your Self-analysis When You Wake Up

We are more critical of ourselves in the afternoon and evening when our brain slows down and fatigue sets in. This means you're more likely to be negative, feel blue and become tearful if you start looking for the meaning of life before you go to bed.

25 Give In To It

Go on, sometimes a girl's got to have a blue day. If you need or want to feel depressed, lie down, curl up and have a good cry, but make sure you resolve to make tomorrow a much better day than today.

chapter 6
Stress busting

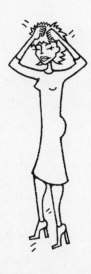

Whether it's coming from your personal relationships, bank manager, work life, family or friends, the fact is that hassle – otherwise known by that favourite buzz word, stress – can't help but get you down. Tired, miserable and headachy? It must be stress. Unable to sleep, fed up with your boyfriend and always crying? It's stress again. Prone to hangovers, bad eating habits and smoking? Well, you'd be healthier if you weren't so stressed, wouldn't you? Or would you?

Actually, stress in itself isn't a bad thing. It's a normal biological and physiological reaction to everyday situations. It's there to help motivate us to do essential things, get us off the couch when we're being lazy and respond to physical danger. Without it we wouldn't have the sense to run for it when something or someone threatens us, or the impetus to get going for an important interview or exam.

As for bad stress, well that's pretty unavoidable too. Maybe you have work projects up to your eyeballs, a boyfriend who keeps threatening to leave, bills you need to pay, a car that keeps breaking down, a bank statement you dare not open and parents about to visit for a week. Not surprising, then, that all you want to do is give in to the lazy way – drink wine, eat pizza and lie on your sofa for the rest of your life. The trouble is that many of us actively use stress as an excuse to avoid taking control of our lives. You can get yourself into a vicious circle of being stressed, incorporating bad habits to cope with the stress – which equals more stress, and leads to more bad habits, and so on and so on. Eventually, the process is guaranteed to leave you feeling like a burnt-out, bloated sofa beast. A bit of an exaggeration perhaps – but you get the drift.

If you have too much stress in your life and never work towards reducing or managing it, you'll feel the following:

- Tired
- Depressed
- Anxious
- Panic ridden
- Tearful
- Hopeless
- Ill
- Angry all the time
- Resentful
- Over-sensitive to criticism

Let it overcome you on a permanent basis and you're likely to suffer from a myriad of health conditions such as:

- Migraines
- Headaches
- Skin rashes
- Stomach upsets
- Insomnia
- Irregular periods
- Ringing in your ears
- Sweating
- Lump in the throat

- Palpitations
- Trembling
- Chest pain
- Nausea
- Diarrhoea
- Sexual problems
- Dizziness
- Tension in the neck
- Irritable Bowel Syndrome

This thing called stress

Stress is not an imaginary ailment but the body's 'fight or flight' response, which is triggered when we perceive a situation, person and/or event as potentially threatening. When this happens, hormones are released from the brain, including adrenalin, which race around the body through the bloodstream. When the hormones reach the heart, lungs and muscles a particular physiological reaction takes place.

"stress in itself isn't a bad thing."

Symptoms Of The 'Fight or Flight' Response:
- Our heart starts pumping faster
- Our breathing quickens
- Our muscles tense ready for action

- Our vision sharpens
- Our stomach knots
- Our thoughts race
- We start sweating

Unfortunately, as most of us don't need to fight or run away, our bodies stay on red alert, unable to relax and unwind. Tension and anxiety remain in the body and just build and build with each stressful event we encounter, leading to the following:

What your skin is trying to tell you

You may not know when you're stressed to the max, but your skin will, and will show you in the following ways:

- Rosacea, eczema and psoriasis – stress will exacerbate all existing skin conditions
- Hives (urticaria), skin rashes and sweat rashes. These are caused by your sweat glands becoming over-productive or by chemical changes in the body, and are all spurred on by stress
- More dandruff – it's caused by increased inflammation of the hair follicles, a by-product of tension
- Acne – stress increases the activity of your sebaceous glands
- Dark circles under your eyes – caused by lack of sleep and the body diverting your blood flow away from unnecessary areas to vital organs
- Wrinkles – frown lines across the forehead, between the eyebrows and around the mouth are a common result of tension and anxiety

What your hair is trying to tell you

Grey hair

Although there is little scientific evidence to back this up, some experts believe that when you're stressed, the body uses up your vitamin B stocks in the body. And as there is a connection between vitamin B depletion and greying hair, you're likely to see a change of hair colour.

Hair loss

Most of us have about 100,000 hairs and we lose about 100 of them a day. If you are losing more than this (i.e. a comb full of hair), it might be due to stress, as hair growth is halted when the body is ill or traumatised. What usually happens is that you go through a stressful event, which at the time makes your hair stop growing, and about eight weeks later you notice more hair loss than usual. The hair will start growing again naturally, but if you're worried, see your GP to rule out other conditions such as an iron deficiency.

What your stomach is trying to tell you

Grumbly stomachs are often caused by stress:

Diarrhoea. Anxiety is one of the commonest causes of the runs

Abdominal pains. These cramps are caused by the stomach muscles clenching and not relaxing

Constipation. It's a by-product of IBS (irritable bowel syndrome), whereby the intestines become more sensitive. IBS also causes diarrhoea, bloating, excess wind and nausea

Irregular periods. Worry and stress can throw off your menstrual cycle or change its duration

Finding it hard to swallow? Feeling a lump in your throat as you swallow or when something stressful happens is a common sign of emotional stress

What your mind is trying to tell you

1. Headaches

Tension Headaches

Location:	a squeezing discomfort on both sides of the temples, like having a tight elastic band round your head
Duration:	several hours
Result of:	depression, anxiety and the contractions of the muscles of the scalp, face and neck
Solution:	massage your scalp and get a regular neck and back massage to avoid the tightening of neck and shoulder muscles

Cluster headaches

Location:	a piercing pain on one side of your head, sometimes behind the eye area
Duration:	a few minutes to a few hours. These usually occur in the early morning or during the night
Result of:	dehydration and stress

tips

Think of your favourite place in the world, then close your eyes and imagine yourself there, relaxed and happy. Do this twice a day for 10 minutes and you'll be calm and stress-free.

Solution: avoid alcohol, smoking, tea and coffee, and never miss a meal as low blood sugar can cause headaches

Sinus headaches

Location: pressure and congestion above the bridge of the nose, causing a dull ache

Duration: a few hours to a couple of days

Result of: a build-up of pressure in the facial sinuses thanks to stress, a cold, flu or working in a dry environment

Solution: nose drops can improve drainage in the sinuses

Migraines

Location: severe headaches which give you a pain on one side of the head and can sometimes extend into the neck and behind the eye. You will feel nauseous and have disturbed vision

Duration: several hours to two to three days

Result of: the expansion and narrowing of blood vessels in the head, triggered by serotonin, a hormone-like substance produced in the blood. The warning signs of a migraine may include tiredness, food craving and blurred vision. Possible triggers are stress, chocolate, hard cheeses, caffeine, red wine and citrus fruits

Solutions: Try the following:

- Lying in a darkened room away from bright lights and loud noise
- Identifying your triggers (so that you can avoid them in future)

- Using your migraines as a way of assessing how stressed you are, and how much stress you can cope with
- Eating small, frequent meals so your blood sugar doesn't dip
- Working out ways you can learn to relax, like yoga and meditation
- An alternative treatment such as acupuncture

2. Anxiety and panic attacks

One in 20 women suffer from anxiety or panic attacks. Factors that increase the likelihood of panic attacks are:

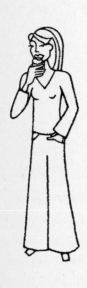

- High levels of stress
- A hectic lifestyle
- A constant state of anxiousness
- A perfectionist streak
- Overwhelming commitments
- Worry
- Alcohol
- Low blood sugar

It's believed that panic attacks are a response to extreme stress and anxiety and occur when a person has been living with high levels of stress for a long time. It's bad news for your mind and body because it means you're living with a high level of tension in your life.

Symptoms of a panic attack

When the body's 'fight or flight' response to perceived danger is left on red alert all the time, you may feel the following:

- A sweaty and cold feeling when something unplanned or potentially worrying happens
- Claustrophobia in crowded, hot and/or noisy places
- Nausea and dizziness
- Heart palpitations
- Over breathing (when you can't catch your breath)
- A ringing in your ears
- An overwhelming sense of doom and terror
- Pins and needles
- Fear of losing control
- Diarrhoea

Experts have found that the people most likely to suffer from panic attacks are those who can't relax – people who are overly self-critical, perfectionist and who bombard themselves with 'shoulds' and 'musts'. The kind of lifestyle you lead also ups your chances:

- Are you overcome with the strains of juggling a job, relationship and friends?
- Do you eat badly and rob yourself of a good night's sleep?
- Are you constantly worried that you're going to lose control of your life?
- Do you worry that if you stop and relax, your world will fall apart?

Another possible trigger for panic attacks is a major life change. Some people experience their first panic attack after something important has happened to them – moving house, getting into debt, breaking up with a partner or the death of a loved one. These will all affect your ability to cope.

Help Yourself By:

- Acknowledging you have the power to control your panic and its causes
- Making better lifestyle choices
- Reassuring yourself that a panic attack isn't life-threatening (it just feels that way)
- Realising your thoughts have a powerful impact on your feelings and behaviour
- Looking at what is happening in your life. Do you feel trapped and stuck? Do you find it difficult to express your feelings?
- Seeing a counsellor for help
- If you're having a panic attack: cupping your hands or holding a paper bag over your nose and mouth and breathing into it for 10 minutes. This will raise levels of carbon dioxide in the bloodstream and relieve symptoms
- Seeing your doctor for advice about drugs that can help to alleviate the panic. There are a number of different types of medication which have proved useful in blocking panic attacks and decreasing anxiety – ask your GP for advice

tips

If you're having a panic attack, cup your hands or hold a paper bag over your nose and mouth and breathing into it for 10 minutes. This will raise levels of carbon dioxide in the bloodstream and relieve symptoms.

What your sleep patterns are trying to tell you

An inability to sleep is primarily caused by stress, and not just internal stress or the worrying kind, but also external stresses such as drinking too much and partying too hard. Not looking at how you stress yourself out will lessen your ability to cope with life, lower your IQ, lower your concentration levels, ruin your relationships and have you sobbing by Friday afternoon. This is because our bodies NEED sleep in order to work effectively and productively.

Throughout the night our bodies follow a sleep pattern. The first 90–100 minutes are non-REM sleep – essential to boost our energy levels after being awake for 16–17 hours. REM sleep, which happens later in the night, is a stage of vigorous brain activity, and plays a major role in boosting our sexual and learning functions and general performance. Do yourself out of either and you're asking for trouble.

Factors That Increase Insomnia:
- Erratic sleep patterns
- Heavy meals
- High alcohol intake
- Coffee
- Worry
- Not taking time to relax during the day
- A highly stressed lifestyle

Experts agree that the way to avoid all of the above, get some sleep and wake up happy, is to take responsibility for your lifestyle. Cut down on your stress, eat properly, work out how much sleep you need to feel full of energy and make sure you get it every night. Try going to bed for a full eight hours for one whole week. If you wake up rested and alert, that's how much you need. If not, decrease by half an hour or add half an hour to see the difference.

How to get a good night's sleep

- Don't watch TV in bed. Watching action or drama films puts your body on red alert and hinders sleep
- Think about your problems an hour before you go to bed and then relax in a hot bath, so your mind is not racing as you try to sleep
- If you can't sleep, get up after 20 minutes and do something until you feel tired
- Don't eat foods that are difficult to digest after 8 pm
- Try alternative therapies, such as the herb valerian, which aids sleep
- Think about seeing someone to discuss your worries

Instant stress relief

Picture the scene – it's 3 pm, you're feeling tired thanks to a heavy, alcohol-fuelled lunch. To make matters

"hold the black coffee and don't reach for that Mars bar."

worse, your boss drops a large file into your lap and suggests you work late. Your best friend calls up hysterical because her boyfriend has dumped her and your mum calls to say your cat's gone missing. Worse still, your thighs seem to have expanded since breakfast, and payday is over a week away. Stressed and in need of a quick fix? Well, hold the black coffee and don't reach for that Mars Bar – here's how to feel better fast:

Breathe deeply

When we're stressed our breathing tends to become shallow, which means our bodies don't get enough oxygen, energy levels flag and we start to yawn more (in order to suck in more oxygen). Practise good breathing – push your stomach out as you breathe in, feel your lungs fill up, and contract your stomach as you breathe out for a count of four. Do this eight times and you'll feel refreshed.

Snack

Preferably on something that will give you energy without a blood sugar high and low. Try a banana, nuts, carrots, or toast and peanut butter for a steady and more effective boost to your energy levels. Drink herbal tea if you can bear it or, if you have to, a milky cup of coffee.

Walk

Preferably outside your office. Air conditioning, stuffy atmospheres, other people's moods and stresses can all affect your energy and concentration levels. Go for a 10-minute walk (without your mobile phone) and you'll instantly feel better, calmer and more able to deal with the hassle around you.

Prioritise

Don't panic. List all the stresses you have and then work out which you can solve immediately, which can be dealt with later and what has to be dealt with on a long-term basis. Now visualise a calm scene – you may not be into the mind-over-matter scene but focusing on calmness and imagining everything at a more peaceful level will slow your heartbeat, halt your panic and help you to focus on solving your stresses.

Long-term lazy stress management

Are you a chronic worrier? Angry all the time, resentful, anxious and/or a guilt addict? If so, you're lowering your immune system, hindering your mental health and generally making your life harder than it needs to be. Help yourself by incorporating some stress management into your life.

Step one: get a grip on your worrying

Living in 'What if ... ' land is a waste of energy, as is pondering on past events and stressing about the future. Become present-orientated and externally motivated, i.e. live in the present and stop thinking so much.

Step two: don't pile up your anger

Okay, so you don't like confrontation, but this doesn't mean you have to swallow all the wrongs being done to you. Speak up and talk about how you feel, or you run the risk of becoming depressed, miserable and put upon. Worse still, you might turn into a passive aggressive – someone who is too passive to argue about what's really bothering them so is argumentative about the small, annoying stuff.

Step three: say no

Don't take on more than you can handle – otherwise known as saying NO! If you overload yourself with responsibilities, you'll feel as if you're living on the edge and come close to burnout. Before saying yes to anything, ask yourself – do you want to do this or do you just feel you *should*?

Step four: don't take on everyone

Stop taking responsibility for everyone else. It's not your fault that someone you know and/or love is unhappy, pathetic or needy. Listen, be a good friend, but don't let them take over your life.

Step five: eat wisely

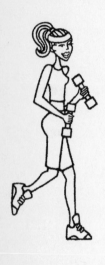

If you feel super-stressed don't turn to alcohol, junk food and cigarettes for help. All they will do is cause mood swings and tiredness, make you feel depressed and anxious, and boost tension levels.

Step six: learn to relax

This doesn't mean going to sleep or lying on the sofa. It means actively relaxing: taking time out from your life, getting a massage, learning to meditate, seeing a counsellor, and/or exercising all release tension and help you to relax.

Step seven: ask for help

No man is an island and all that jazz – so don't think you have to do everything on your own because (a) you don't have to, and (b) what are you proving if you do?

Step eight: live it up

As they say, you only come by this way once, so what are you waiting for? This doesn't mean forgoing all stress and going back to lazy-girl status, but living your life fully and actively without putting yourself under pressure to work harder, earn more and do all the things everyone tells you you're supposed to.

Step nine: be realistic

Even the best-laid plans go to pot, so there's no point freaking out if life doesn't go the way you want, or whining about the unfairness of it all. Learn to go with the flow – you won't be sorry.

Step ten: try yoga

Especially when things get tough. Studies show that 80 % of us don't breathe properly. To learn to breathe properly all the time, try doing a form of exercise that focuses on breathing. Yoga, Pilates and Tai Chi are all perfect for stress relief and ridding the body of tension and anxiety.

Step eleven: get the balance right

All work and no play will make you ultra-stressed. All play and no work will have the same effect only the stresses will be different. For less hassle, make sure your life has an equal balance of work, play, socialising and private downtime.

"don't take everything so seriously."

Step twelve: lighten up

Don't take everything so seriously – you'll be surprised how much happier you'll be.

25 ways to bust stress

1 Have A Hot Bath
Soak in a hot bath for 20 minutes. Not only will your muscles relax and let go of tension, the heat will also lower your blood pressure by encouraging your blood vessels to dilate.

2 Put Some Ice On Your Head
It's one of the fastest ways to stop a headache and relieve tension. Place ice in a towel, lay it on your forehead or on the base of your neck and relax.

3 Fill Up Your Lungs
Take a deep breath and count to six as you release. This will help you relax and unwind. But don't do this for more than five breaths or you'll feel lightheaded.

4 Visualise Your Way To Inner Peace
Think of your favourite place in the world, then close your eyes and imagine yourself there, relaxed and happy. Do this twice a day for 10 minutes (on the bus, on the floor, at work) and you'll be calm and stress-free.

5 Get Creative
Being under-stressed is as much a problem as being over-stressed. Lack of stimulation is a depressant and likely to leave you feeling lonely and isolated. To avoid this you need to immerse yourself in something new that involves using your brain creatively.

6 Get A Massage
Massage has been shown to be a great stress reliever, especially if you're overloaded with responsibilities. It releases tension and anxiety and, at the same time, helps you to relax and slows down your heartbeat.

7 Lie On The Sofa
Downtime of 10–30 minutes on the sofa with the phone switched off is an excellent form of stress management. It will help you recharge your batteries and cope with external pressures in your life.

8 Go Outside
Sometimes a girl just has to get

away from her problems. Twenty minutes of fresh air and sunshine will not only improve your breathing and help you relax, it will also re-energise you.

9 Take A Holiday

A major study in the US found that people who hadn't taken a holiday in two years were more likely to suffer stress-related illnesses and eventual burnout. Take time off once every four months for optimum benefit.

10 Live In The Moment (But Plan For Tomorrow)

You'll not only have fun, you'll get more done, worry less, and keep your stress in perspective.

11 Don't Be A Drama Queen

Exaggerating your problems and past disasters to friends and family just makes you relive the stress over and over. The aim is to learn from what's happened, not make a movie out of it.

12 Have Sex

Researchers have found sex reduces tension and promotes deep and restful sleep because endorphins are released by sexual stimulation.

13 Don't Be A Tech Junkie

Emails, mobiles, telephones, faxes, text messages – it's good to stay in touch but not so good if you're obsessed.

14 See Someone Professional

This is essential if you are on the brink of despair, cry every day and suffer from anxiety or panic attacks. Look for a professional counsellor/therapist who can help you weave your way through the stresses and strains of your life (see BAC in Resources and talk to your GP).

15 Do Something You're Scared Of Once A Month

Whether it's joining a gym, roller-blading, salsa dancing or asking someone out, it will boost your self-confidence, double your self-esteem and help you put your problems in perspective.

16 Give Yourself A Break

Okay, so you're not the fittest, thinnest, smartest person out there but who cares? You don't have to be!

17 Get A Strategy
Or else life and all its stresses will just take over. Write a list of 10 things you want from life, maybe to buy a house, get fit, go out more, have a holiday, meet someone etc., and then think about how you're going to get there and start working towards it.

18 Be More Sociable
Especially if you're feeling down. Laugh more, ease up on yourself and off-load some of your stresses with supportive friends, and it will help you forget your problems for the night.

19 Say What You Mean
The fastest way to get stressed-out is to say, 'It's fine', when it's not. Learn to stand up for yourself and what you believe in and you won't be in danger of internal stress overload.

20 Take Responsibility For Your Health
Studies show that looking after your health will not only make you feel happier but will stop you stressing about your body image and boost your self-esteem.

21 Cuddle Someone (Or Something)
Cuddling or stroking is a fast way to lower your stress levels and boost your feelings of wellbeing.

22 Don't Relive Your Past
Weird but true – rehashing stressful events won't make you feel better but will only make you stressed all over again. Rather than reliving the stress, write it down, tear it up and then rip it into small pieces and throw it away. Symbolic, maybe, but it will send the right message to your brain.

23 Talk About It
Better out than in when it comes to problems and the blues.

24 Rest Up At Weekends
Believe your mother when she tells you not to keep burning the candle at both ends.

25 Be Realistic
You're not aiming for a stress-free existence, just better management of your stress levels.

chapter 7
Looks

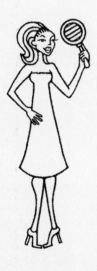

Your face is your fortune, or so they say, but it won't be if you live it up so much that you end up looking 40 when you're still 25! If you're not a follower of the always-wear-sunscreen, cleanse, tone, moisturise, never-pick-your-spots and drink-lots-of-water brigade – it's likely that: (1) you rarely look in the mirror, (2) age and bad living hasn't caught up with you yet, or (3) you're blessed with good genes.

The bad news is that your lifestyle will eventually catch up with your face and it will happen sooner than you think. But you don't have to become beauty obsessed to keep the signs of ageing at bay. There are plenty of ways to maximise your looks that don't involve going down either the plastic-surgery or brown-paper-bag path. The key to looking good isn't to focus in on your looks and become a product-junkie, but to get yourself a health regime which will not only improve your lifestyle but, as a natural by-product, also improve your looks.

What's ageing you?

While genes and biological factors account for much of the way you age, you can speed up the process with lazy living. Here's how:

Your stress levels

Too much stress in your life not only ups your chances of high blood pressure and heart disease, it also gives you wrinkles. Anxiety uses up vital nutrients and slows down cellular turnover.

Your suncare routine

Research shows that 95% of skin ageing is caused by sunlight. While studies indicate that men are more likely to end up with wrinkles than women (that old macho thing about not using sun cream), take his advice and you'll look the same!

Your diet

After the age of 30 you can't get away with a sedentary lifestyle and an unhealthy diet. Eat rubbish all day and you can expect any of the following to set in by the time you're 45: muscle wasting, weak bones, general lethargy and a whole multitude of age-related diseases such as athero-sclerosis (hardening of the arteries).

Your weight

Thanks to a slower metabolism and substantial muscle loss after the age of 30, women gain on average almost 5 kg (11lbs) between the ages of 35 and 45, and one more between 45 and 55. If you want to avoid this you have to eat more healthily, and move more.

The lazy girl's guide to staying young and beautiful

Have glowing skin

For fantastic skin you don't need to spend a fortune at a cosmetics counter, have surgery or buy the most expensive lotion or potion on the market – you just need to feed your face. Certain vitamins stimulate the skin and help with the formation of new skin cells. The ones to focus on are A, C and E – the antioxidants.

- Vitamin A regulates the way your body grows and develops. It's essential for healthy skin, as well as teeth and nails. Natural sources include carrots, oily fish, cheese, milk, spinach and eggs
- Vitamin C is essential for the production of collagen, the support mechanism of your skin. Without it, the scaffolding below your cheeks literally falls down. Vitamin C is found in green leafy vegetables, herbs and fruit such as strawberries, mangoes and citrus fruit
- Vitamin E strengthens muscle fibres and improves skin suppleness, helping your cheeks to maintain that bouncy exterior. Food sources include avocado, eggs, nuts and seeds, wholemeal pasta and soya milk

Skin myths

Myth: *Sleeping in your make up is bad for you*
Well, it's bad for your sheets and it's not so attractive in the morning, but it's not the worst thing you can do to your skin. After all, the make up has been on your face all day, and how does your skin know it's bedtime? – meaning it won't harm your skin either way. However, forget to cleanse in the morning and keep layering it on and you're asking for a skin breakout.

Myth: *It's essential to cleanse, tone and moisturise*
Rumour has it that this 'beauty law' was made up by the make up companies to ensure you bought more of their products. Whether you believe it or not, one thing's for

"you can't change your skin from the outside."

sure, plenty of women get by without doing all of the above. The simple fact is that you can't change your skin from the outside, and all these products do is buff the skin and make it appear more glowing.

Myth: *Creams can re-hydrate your skin*
Also untrue. If your skin is dehydrated, you are dehydrated. No amount of expensive creams will make your skin more moist. Drink more fluids and your skin will improve.

Myth: *Face creams can get rid of your wrinkles*
Nothing can get rid of your wrinkles (except surgery). What most 'miracle' creams do is plump up the skin so your wrinkles appear to disappear for a while.

Myth: *Wrinkles are avoidable*
Sadly not! As we age our skin gets thinner and the tissues that hold the skin together naturally loosen and sag. If you frown a lot, smoke, squint in the sun and laugh, you can expect some furrows. If your parents are wrinkly, you will be too – it's in the genes. Is it worth worrying about? No, because everyone you know will have them by the time you do.

Hold on to your hair
Like your skin, your hair is a natural indicator of how

healthy you are. The average human head has approximately 100,000 strands of hair and we usually lose between 75 and 100 of these each day. It sounds a lot but new ones replace most of it. If you find you are suffering from accelerated hair loss, it could be down to the way you're living your life – bad diet, too much stress, and hormone problems all stop your hair from growing. The good news is that glossy, healthy hair doesn't have to be something you only see in magazines. Act on the following and you'll have flowing locks in no time:

- Think about the stress you're under. Chronic stress can wreak havoc on your hair. This is because stress causes the muscles to constrict and triggers tension in the scalp. It can also make existing hair problems such as dryness, dandruff or a greasy scalp worse
- Avoid harsh hair treatments. Chemical treatments and over-colouring can break and split your hair, as can vigorous drying with a hairdryer. Hair loses about a third of its natural moisture when it's blown dry
- Look for grey bits. People go grey when the production of melanin (the pigment that gives hair its colour) stops. If this is already happening to you, blame stress levels. High levels of anxiety disrupt the flow of blood and nutrients to the hair follicles. Illness, bad diet and depression can also affect the production of melanin, causing both men and women to end up with prematurely grey hair
- Load up on vitamins. For shiny, healthy hair, bolster your diet

with foods rich in zinc and vitamin A (seafood, nuts and green leafy vegetables), and also B$_6$ (eggs and wholemeal bread), which helps sustain the production of new hair

Hair myths

Myth: *You need to wash it every day*
Not true – hair only needs to be washed every two to three days, sometimes less. Do it more often and you're washing out natural oils.

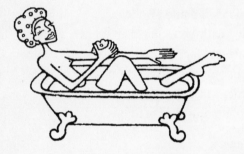

Myth: *You don't need to protect it in the sun*
You do if you want to maintain its condition. Use shampoos and/or sprays that contain a UV filter, and if in doubt, wear a hat. On post-sun days, you'll need a conditioner to bring it back to life.

Myth: *You shouldn't pull your hair*
You shouldn't pull it when you're stressed, but if you massage your scalp and gently pull your hair for two minutes every day, you'll boost circulation and promote hair growth.

Say goodbye to spots

Acne, pimples, zits, call them what you may, the truth is they are not just the scourge of the average teenager. If you're prone to spots, especially near your period, they may be being triggered by male hormones known as androgens, which control oil production in the body. Usually the body's tiny oil sebaceous glands produce enough lubrication (known as sebum) to keep the skin smooth and make hair shine. However, when these glands overproduce, the excess oil causes the hair follicle ducts to shed their lining too quickly, and dead skin cells begin to block up your skin pores. Once plugged, the duct becomes inflamed with bacteria and swells, until the surface of the skin above it becomes red and swollen.

If you can't live with your skin any longer, The Acne Support Group suggests applying the two-month rule to any acne treatment you try. If you do not see a 35–50% marked improvement in your skin after eight weeks, you should try a different course of action.

1. Self-medication.

Buy a product with the active ingredient benzoyl peroxide. This works on acne by reducing sebum production from the skin's oil glands and drying out the skin. Always start with a low dosage, i.e. 2.5% of this ingredient, and then move up to a larger dose, as it can burn the skin. If that has no effect, try a different product, this time with the active ingredient azelaic acid. This substance can kill bacteria, and unblock plugged-up hair follicles by loosening blackheads.

2. Oral antibiotics

If you have scarring from your spots (caused by a spot being so

tips

To zap spots with products always allow eight weeks for results to show.

deep in the hair follicle that it pushed the skin up and eventually caused a crater), see your GP for advice. Four oral antibiotic treatments are available for acne: tetracycline, doxycycline, minocycline and erythromycin. They can take up to six months to work, so you need to persevere.

3. Dermatologists and Roaccutane (Isoretinoin)

Roaccutane has been available in the UK for 15 years and in the States for 20 years. This drug is only available on prescription from a hospital dermatologist (you need to be referred by your GP) and is only used on patients who have severe acne and on those who have tried several courses of antibiotics. Roaccutane has revolutionised the treatment of severe acne as it is the only drug available that works on all its aspects: it helps to dry up excess oil, stop sebum production, reduce inflammation and subsequent scarring. Seventy-five per cent of people who take this drug do not have a relapse.

Spot myths

Myth: *You can't pick your spots*
Well, you're not supposed to, but you can if you're desperate. If you're going to squeeze, use two tissues and the sides of your fingers. Don't squeeze inwards but pull the skin apart away from the centre and the spot should 'pop'.

Myth: *Spots are caused by chocolate and fatty foods like chips*
A lie perpetrated by your parents to stop you eating all

the Milk Tray. Spots are not caused by anything you eat and drink, including chocolate. This is one of life's great untruths.

Myth: *The sun is good for your spots*
The sun can dry out spots but it has a very short-term effect – long-term exposure will only dry your skin out and do more damage than any spot ever could.

Myth: *Spots are caused by dirty skin*
Also untrue – blackheads aren't bits of dirt, but trapped sebum (oil), which has turned dark in the air.

Myth: *Toothpaste can zap a spot*
The fluoride in toothpaste can't kill off the bacteria in spots – so don't even bother to try this one.

Super suncare

"skin cancer and skin damage can happen to anyone."

Research shows that sunbathing is literally the kiss of death, yet a new study shows that one in four of us strips down without protection the second the sun comes out. Seventy-one per cent of us still think a tan looks healthy and 60% of us still want to feel the burn. Little wonder, then, that cases of skin cancer have doubled in the UK in the past 20 years. Of course, skin cancer and skin damage can happen to anyone. However, you're at a higher risk of developing skin cancer if you:

- Have fair hair with a tendency to freckle
- Regularly get sunburnt and sit out in the sun
- Have light eyes and blond or red hair
- Use no sunscreen or protection that's under SPF 15
- Have a family history of skin cancer (the risk is 50% greater if you have two close relatives who have had melanoma)
- Have more than five large moles (over 5 mm across)
- Notice new moles appearing on your skin
- Regularly use sunbeds

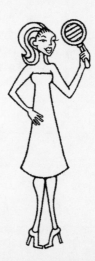

How to protect yourself

You don't have to avoid the sun to stay safe (after all it's an essential source of vitamin D), but if you're a sun lizard, it's essential you protect yourself:

- Always wear a sunscreen with a protection factor of SPF 15 – and apply it 20 minutes before you go out so you don't sweat it off
- Avoid the sun between 11 am and 3 pm as that's when it's at its strongest
- Even intermittent trips into the sun can cause damage – so protect your skin during your lunch hour
- Think about a sunscreen for your hair and a hat – your hair won't protect your scalp from getting burnt
- Apply more sunscreen to your face than to the rest of your body
- Reapply sunscreen every 2–3 hours, or when you feel your skin tingling
- If you do go out, help yourself by covering up with loose cotton clothes, a hat, sunglasses and UV protection
- Check your skin regularly for changes in moles, new moles or bumps
- Wear sunglasses – exposure of the eye area to the sun contributes to decreasing vision as you get older

Suncare myths

Myth: *Sunbeds won't damage your skin*

Thinking about hopping on a sunbed because you've read it's safer for you? Well, think again – the UV rays you absorb on a sunbed are nearly twenty times stronger than the sun's rays. Also, contrary to popular belief, the UVA rays produced by sunbeds are not harmless, and can actually cause deeper damage to the skin than the sun. A 30-minute roast on a bed equals an entire day of sun on the beach. Solution – fake it!

Myth: *Your make up is SPF 15 and you always wear a t-shirt so you're fine*
A t-shirt only provides an SPF of 5–9 so you also need sunscreen. The SPF in make up isn't as effective as sunscreen because you don't apply as much. Plus, some products only protect against UVB rays and not UVAs.

Myth: *You only need to apply once a day*
You need to reapply sun cream every two hours. And don't be fooled into thinking you can decrease the protection factor as the summer goes on. The skin does not become resilient to UV rays.

Myth: *You always sit in the shade so you don't need sunscreen*
A shaded umbrella – just like sand, water and the pavement – will reflect 85% of the sun's rays back onto your skin, so slap on the cream.

Myth: *It's the UK – you don't need to wear sunscreen*
One in five of us won't wear sun protection because it's just 'too much hassle'. Scary statistics considering cases of malignant melanoma amongst the under 30s have risen

tips

If you're determined to expose yourself to the sun, use a sunscreen that ensures you won't burn as this will lower your risk of damaging your skin for good.

by 70%! The sun in the UK is as strong as the sun in Europe – you may think it's not going to damage your skin but it will, even on a cloudy day.

Myth: *I'm always inside at work so I don't need a sunscreen* An American study found that the average office worker gets around 15 hours of accidental sun exposure a week while nipping out on errands, walking to work and sitting in the sun at lunch, so you do need sunscreen.

Myth: *I'm working on a safe tan* There's no such thing – any change in skin colour is a sign of skin damage. If you're determined to do it, use a sunscreen that ensures you won't burn as this will lower your risk of damaging your skin for good.

Water your body

Sixty per cent of us drink less than half our recommended daily allowance of water, which means most of us are de-hydrated. This is bad news for your body, because it's the first place the body sucks moisture from when it's in need. Forget to reboot your water stocks and you're asking for dry skin, the energy levels of someone twice your age, and bags under your eyes. Water also hydrates our organs, cushions the nervous system and is essential for joints, eyes and the digestive system. Without it we're asking for piercing headaches, problems with concentration, bad breath, mood swings and extreme tiredness.

Help Yourself By:

- Drinking before you get thirsty – the body's thirst receptors only kick in as you become dehydrated. If you're not sure whether you need more water, take a look at your urine. The darker the colour the more dehydrated you are, and the more water you need to drink. If the thought of guzzling 10 glasses a day is too much for you, think of it as half a glass of water every half an hour, and you'll easily hit your quota

- Thinking about when you need more water. Long-distance travellers in particular need to pay attention to how much water they drink. Post-flight dehydration, which manifests itself as headaches, constipation, aches and pains, is common because flying exacerbates dehydration

- Drinking two extra glasses of water for every cup of coffee or glass of wine

- Keeping alcohol to a minimum – for every 1 ml of alcohol, 10 ml is lost in urine and fluids. Alcohol also acts as a diuretic, which means it tricks your body into over-urinating, leading to exaggerated fluid loss

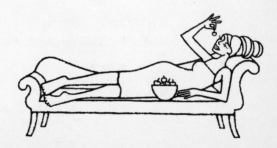

Drink more water and . . .

- The condition of your skin will improve
- You'll have more energy
- You'll lose weight (research shows that people often eat when their energy levels are low when they really just need a drink)
- Your digestive system will work better
- You'll sleep better
- You'll feel less hungry
- Your eyes will be brighter
- You'll have less joint pain
- You'll avoid gallstones
- You'll reduce your risk of cancer of the colon

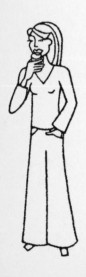

Water myths

Myth: *You don't need water because you drink other things*
Tea, fruit juices and vegetables all contain water and you consume lots of these. Yes, but your water requirement is in addition to all these things. Plus, tea is a diuretic, so you actually lose fluid when you drink it.

Myth: *Bottled water is better for you*
Untrue – studies show that tap water is the cleanest water you can get, so you've no excuse not to drink it.

Myth: *You don't like the taste*
Water doesn't actually taste of anything so what you're missing is the taste of chemicals and sugar.

Look after your teeth

Thanks to lower levels of tooth decay, 90% of us can now expect to keep our teeth for life. However, while false teeth may be a thing of the past, maintaining a bright white smile as our teeth get older and more worn and yellowed is not so easy. Teeth start to yellow because the enamel gets thinner – and so more of the inside of the tooth shows through.

You may not particularly care what your teeth look like, but studies show that they can and will affect your chances in life and in your career. According to research, when you meet someone you look first into their eyes, and then at their teeth. Quite simply, white, uniformed teeth give the impression of beauty and youth, and grubby, stained, irregular ones don't. Things that can stain your teeth are:

- Cigarettes
- Antibiotics
- Red wine
- Coffee
- Bad cleaning technique

Fortunately, even if you're too lazy to look after your teeth properly, your dentist can remove the small stains in around 20 minutes. Teeth whitening, another useful technique, is usually carried out over the course of three weeks and the effects last up to seven years.

As far as your gums are concerned, you should aim at

having pink, healthy-looking ones – not ones that bleed or give off an odour when you floss. This means brush twice a day, preferably with an electric toothbrush, floss daily and see your dentist every six months.

Help Yourself By:

- Brushing twice a day
- Flossing once a day
- Visiting the dentist every six months

Teeth myths

Myth: *Fillings last for ever*
Sadly not. If you have a mouth full of old fillings from childhood you should go and get them checked. If they are cracked, decay inside your tooth could be causing irreversible damage.

Myth: *White fillings are better*
You can have your old silver amalgam fillings replaced by white fillings, but the improvement will only be aesthetic. While white fillings are effective and long lasting in most cases, they do not work well in deep fillings.

Healthy Nails

If you're in good health, your nails will be shiny with a smooth surface. The plate, i.e. the main part of the nail, will look pink and the nail will be strong, not brittle.

Diet is the most important thing when it comes to

healthy nails. A diet lacking in essential minerals, like iron, calcium and zinc, will make them brittle and flaky. Other factors that work against your nails are:

- Too much alcohol – it robs your body of the essential nutrients needed to make healthy nails
- Strong soaps – they can cause flaking and splitting

Help Yourself By:
- Eating more dairy products, spinach, dried apricots and oily fish and seafood
- Cutting your nails rather than biting them off, which makes them prone to flaking

Nail myths

Myth: *White marks on the nail are a sign of calcium deficiency*
Actually, white marks are signs of nail damage – caused by bumps to the base of the nail as it was growing (a fifth of the nail is hidden under the skin, at the base of the nail plate).

Don't Forget Your Feet

Want bare-able feet? Then start by looking after them. Chiropodists say that the feet are the most neglected area of the body, and yet they're also the part that takes all the weight (literally).

For Healthy Feet:

- Go barefoot more often. It will help exercise the 26 bones and 20 muscles that make up your foot
- Walk heel to toe
- Wear comfortable shoes as often as you can. Two in five British women admit to wearing uncomfortable shoes to look good. While one night won't kill you, repeated abuse can lead to bunions, corns and ingrown toenails
- Treat your feet. Especially if you have dried, cracked skin or weird itches. The chances are you have athlete's foot – a fungal infection that could spread. Treat it with over-the-counter products or tea tree oil.

tips

Go barefoot more often. It will help exercise the 26 bones and 20 muscles that make up your foot

25 ways to keep young and beautiful

1 Use Sun Cream With A High SPF
As 95% of skin ageing is caused by sunlight, dermatologists suggest protecting your skin on a daily basis with sun creams and moisturisers with high SPF factors.

2 Exercise
Research at Yale University in the US has shown that exercise helps to delay your body's natural degeneration.

3 Take An Antioxidant
Free radicals (molecules which destroy cells in the body) contribute towards ageing and age-related disease such as osteoarthritis and cardiovascular disease. Damage comes in the form of chemicals ingested in food and drink, sunlight, smoking, pollution, alcohol and pesticides. Take a daily antioxidant to protect yourself.

4 Help Your Hair To Grow
Healthy hair cells, like any other cells in your body, need the right nutrients in order to thrive. Keeping up your zinc, iron and vitamin B12 levels can slow down hair thinning.

5 Have More Cappuccinos
Women need 800 g of calcium a day. Good sources are dairy products, spinach, broccoli and dried fruit. There's lots of calcium in cappuccinos.

6 Have More Sex
Have sex at least twice a week and you'll reduce your risk of premature death by 36%.

7 Laugh More
Laughing ups the production of infection and cancer-fighting cells by 25%.

8 Make New Friends
Research shows people who have large social groups, live longer, stay happier and are less stressed.

9 Have A Good Cry

A good sob is great for your skin and your stress levels. Plus, it leaves you looking younger as it works the muscles in the face and helps them relax.

10 Don't Brush Too Much

This one applies to your teeth and your hair. Brush your teeth too vigorously and you could damage your gums, wear down the enamel and take off that natural shine. Brush your hair too much and you'll be putting excess pressure on the hair root.

11 Avoid Frowning

If you have deep lines in your forehead, a crease around your mouth or lines under your eyes and you're not a sun bunny, you could be a secret frowner. Check your set expression to see if it's a furrowed one. If it is, change it by continually telling yourself to relax. Practise in front of the mirror first and you'll see those lines disappear as you breathe more deeply and let your shoulders drop.

12 Fire Up Your Energy Levels

It's the key to appearing younger. You may feel as if you are on your last legs but if you can fake it, others will assume you're younger than you are and treat you as such.

13 Look After Your Hands

Believe it or not, the skin on your hands is as susceptible to sun damage and extreme weather as your face. To help them stay young and not give away your age, glove them in winter and slap sunscreen on in summer.

14 Breathe Properly

Most of us don't breathe properly. We take breaths that are too shallow and don't use our whole diaphragm, which makes us feel lethargic and tired (we yawn to take in more oxygen). To breathe properly, you should feel your lungs expanding and deflating slowly. A good gulp of oxygen will also do wonders for your skin.

15 Get Your Eyebrows Shaped

Also known as the instant

face-lift as it defines your eyes, makes you look less overgrown and wild, and gives your pupils a wider, clearer look.

16 Use Plenty Of Sun Cream
Okay, so you don't want to look like a big shiny ball, but the truth is that to get effective protection you need to apply at least $2/3$ of a teaspoonful-sized squirt to your face. Don't rub it in, but pat it on top of your skin with your fingertips, or you could actually be rubbing it off.

17 Flirt
If you want to swamp your body with feel-good chemicals, then indulge in at least one flirtation a week. It will combat depression, raise your self-esteem and make you feel more confident about your body.

18 Don't Worry
Worry can age you faster than an afternoon in the sunshine. If you want to look younger and feel happier get yourself an optimistic nature. Don't be a glass-half-empty girl, but a glass-half-full one.

19 Challenge Yourself
Scared your mind and body is going to pot? It could be that you need some challenges to get you going. Studies show that intelligence is enhanced by learning new skills as you progress through life. So keep pushing yourself.

20 Be A Well Woman
Get those essential health checks so you can prevent future illness. Tests to get regularly are: blood cholesterol, blood pressure and a cervical smear. You should also carry out a breast exam on yourself every month, and get checked for STIs if you've had unprotected sex.

21 Protect Your Skin In The Sea
When the skin is dry, 8% of the sun's rays penetrate it, but when it's wet, 38% gets through. This means you need to apply a good dose of sunscreen before and after you go swimming.

22 Avoid Sun Bingeing
Short bursts of sunlight are as

damaging to your skin as long periods – so don't be a lunch-time sun binger.

23 See Yourself As A Healthy Person

Research shows that if you can visualise yourself full of vitality and energy, you'll be able to motivate yourself to end up that way.

24 Snack On Vegetables

This may sound boring and dull but studies show that eating vegetables daily can slow down ageing by as much as 10–15 years. Well worth swapping that crisp packet for some carrots!

25 Don't Let Your Birthdays Hold You Back

If you keep active and live the way you want, whatever your age, you'll stay happier and healthier for longer.

chapter 8
How to be extremely knowledgeable about health (without trying)

By this stage of the book, you should be well on your way to becoming a health goddess – unless, of course, you've acted true to lazy-girl form and haven't read the rest of the book/are reading this over someone's shoulder in a bookstore and/or are hoping you can get away with just reading this chapter.

However you got here, you'll be happy to know that this chapter is guaranteed to give you some fake health kudos. Read it, memorise it and drop it into conversation and no one will ever mention the word lazy in your presence again.

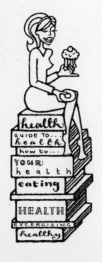

* For super lazy ease, there are two descriptions per entry in the following health glossary – one technical, one summarised.

Acupuncture

Technical version: An ancient technique used to heal various conditions and ailments. Acupuncture involves placing sterilised needles into the skin along the body's energy pathways (meridians) in order to 'clear' problems/ illnesses. It releases the body's natural painkillers and helps 'cure' pain – and scientific studies show that it really does work.

Lazy girl's version: Having needles stuck into your skin isn't the nightmare you might imagine. The needles are not plunged in randomly or deeply. They don't hurt and you won't bleed.

Good For:
- Chronic pain
- PMT
- Fatigue
- Skin conditions
- Nausea

Alexander Technique

Technical version: Postural re-alignment technique that teaches you how to sit, stand, bend and use your spine effectively. Banishes back pain, improves posture and helps with stress, breathing problems and headaches.

Lazy girl's version: The perfect way to learn to walk like a supermodel, and get out of a car without falling onto your face.

Good For:

- Back pain
- Stress
- Persistent headaches
- People who are too lazy to stand up straight

Antioxidants

Technical version: Antioxidants mop up the damage that free radicals (see under f) do to your body. Keep levels of antioxidants high in your body and you'll age more slowly. Antioxidants can be found in brightly coloured vegetables such as tomatoes and peppers, leafy green vegetables, and in fruits with a high vitamin C content.

Lazy girl's version: Your mum wasn't lying when she said those vegetables were good for you – so eat them!

Good For:

- Cancer-fighting properties
- Anti-ageing properties

Aromatherapy

Technical version: The application of various plant essential oils (there are about 400 in total) which, when mixed with a base oil and applied to the skin, supposedly help bring about changes within the body's enzymes and ease conditions such as PMT, IBS, etc.

Lazy girl's version: Nice-smelling oils that can possibly cure everything from mosquito bites to headaches.

Athlete's Foot

Technical version: Fungal infection found between the toes, which makes the skin turn white, soggy and sore. See your pharmacist for an anti-fungal medication.

Lazy girl's version: Wear your trainers too much and your feet will revolt (literally).

Ayurvedic Medicine

Technical version: Ayurveda means 'the science of life' and is a holistic method of treating illnesses. Each patient is assessed via a process that analyses their constitution and lifestyle, rather than just their symptoms. Treatment is given in the form of dietary advice, supplements, massage and meditation.

Lazy girl's version: Trendy Indian alternative medicine based on three body types.

Good For:
- Allergies
- Skin complaints
- Stomach gripes
- PMT
- Headaches

Back Pain

Technical version: Over 70% of people suffer from back pain. In women it's usually due to weak stomach muscles,

tips

Back pain and back posture go hand in hand. Learn to stand and sit properly and your back pain will eventually disappear.

which means that the back muscles have to support both the back and front of the body. While 90% of back pain will get better without treatment, back pain often recurs, in which case it's wise to visit an osteopath (a specialist in the structure of the spine) for an accurate diagnosis and to discuss preventative techniques.

Lazy girl's version: Sort out your posture and work on your abdominal muscles and your back pain will disappear.

Botox Injections

Technical version: Botox, also known as botulinum toxin A, is used to reduce signs of ageing by getting rid of wrinkles and frown lines. The process takes about 10 minutes and involves a cosmetic surgeon injecting minute quantities of Botox into contracted muscles to help smooth them out.

Lazy girl's version: A strand of botulism (yes, the very same culprit behind food poisoning) is injected into your face to paralyse your forehead muscles so you can look unlined, unstressed and forever young.

Good For:

- Frown lines
- Wrinkles
- Currently being tested for use on migraine sufferers

Cellulite

Technical version: Deposits of fat under the skin, which lead to a dimpled look. Cellulite is mainly the result of lifestyle choices and can be lessened by improving your diet, exercise and massage.

Lazy girl's version: Squishy, orange-peel skin on the thighs and bottom. The result of doing all the things you love to do but know you shouldn't.

Cholesterol

Technical version: Cholesterol is essential for a number of bodily functions, such as hormonal balance and digestion. However, a high level of cholesterol in the body can lead to serious health problems and is a major risk factor in heart disease. As it has no symptoms, a blood test is the only way to detect a high cholesterol level. Luckily, once you know you have high cholesterol, it's easy to lower your levels through diet, weight control and drugs.

Lazy girl's version: Cholesterol is the stuff that clogs up your arteries and leads to a heart attack. Eat healthily and you won't die early.

Colonic Irrigation

Technical version: Colonic irrigation is a gentle, internal way of flushing out the bowel. Purified water is pumped through the colon via a tube to help stored faecal matter, gas, mucus and toxic substances flush their way out. Said to be the perfect detox.

Lazy girl's version: A procedure whereby a tube is pushed up your bottom and water poured in and flushed out (as gross as it sounds).

Good For:
- Constipation
- Mental clarity
- Weight problems
- Headaches

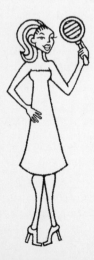

Dandruff

Technical version: Dandruff is thought to be caused by an overgrowth of fungus found normally on the scalp. The fungus causes scales of dead skin to be shed from the scalp in small white bits. It's easily banished with medicated shampoo.

Lazy girl's version: If there's a snowstorm every time you shake your head, you have dandruff.

Deep Vein Thrombosis

Technical version: Deep vein thrombosis is the much talked about long-distance air travel condition caused by the formation of large blood clots in the leg. Under normal everyday conditions, the movement of the calf muscle in the leg pumps blood back to the heart, keeping the circulation in the body going. However, in situations where a person is immobile and/or cramped for a long period of time, such as on a plane, blood can pool and a clot can form in the leg. This clot can later travel to the heart and lungs with fatal consequences. The good news is that the normal risk of DVT in everyday life is about 5 in 100,000 so it's not only the cramped circumstances which make us prone to DVT during a flight, but also pre-existing conditions, such as your age and your health.

Lazy girl's version: Avoid DVT by being careful about how you sit when travelling by plane. Curling up in your seat or crossing your legs will hinder circulation. Your best bet is to walk around and stretch your legs out at least once every half an hour.

Detox

Technical version: Detoxing is a spring-clean system where you limit your diet for a short period of time to water and very basic food in order to rid the body of harmful toxins, which slow your system down. It's usually a two-stage process of cleansing followed by what's known as 'nutritional balancing' ie. learning to eat healthily.

Lazy girl's version: The fruit and vegetable diet that eliminates everything you like to eat. Best done by staying in bed for two days or else you'll feel dizzy, have bad breath and moan to everyone you know.

Good For:
- Brighter skin
- Fatigue
- Weight loss

Dysmenorrhoea

Technical version: The medical name for painful periods. In most women this pain also causes nausea, tiredness, back pain and sometimes headaches. Primary dysmenorrhoea is caused by the release of the hormone prostaglandin in the uterus. Prostaglandin helps propel the womb lining out of your body during your period and works in spasms, hence the cramps. Secondary dysmenorrhoea is a different sort of pain altogether. It lasts longer, has a higher than normal intensity and is caused not by hormones, but by a recognised condition such as uterine fibroids, endo-metriosis, or a pelvic infection.

Lazy girl's version: Period pain.

Eczema

Technical version: Inflammatory skin disease that usually appears on the hands, inside the elbows and behind the knees. Around 1 in 10 people are affected. Eczema runs in families but is also triggered by allergies. Treatment is by steroid creams (prescribed by your GP), herbalism or homeopathy.

Lazy girl's version: Dry, scaly, thickened skin; itching and redness; sometimes blisters.

Flower Remedies (also known as Bach Flower Remedies)

tips

Take Rescue Remedy to calm your nerves before making a speech or taking an exam.

Technical version: Plant remedies which are based on the belief that illnesses are due to emotional stresses and, therefore, in order to treat the ailment you have to treat the stresses. The stresses are divided into: fear, indecision, loneliness, over-sensitivity, despair, overcare and lack of interest. The remedies are all infused from flower heads and come in tincture form. You need to dilute the tincture in water before drinking.

Lazy girl's version: The most popular flower remedy is known as Rescue Remedy and is meant to work wonders if you're nervous, have to make a speech or are suffering from panic attacks. There's no scientific evidence to say it works, but users swear by it.

Good For:

- Panic attacks
- Anxiety
- Pre-exam nerves
- Public speaking
- The blues

Free Radicals

Technical version: Free radicals are molecules that destroy cells in the body. They have been shown to contribute towards ageing and age-related disease such as osteo-arthritis, cancer and cardiovascular disease.

Lazy girl's version: Environmental nasties that will pollute your body if you don't protect yourself by eating more fruit and vegetables.

Genetically Modified (GM) Foods

Technical version: GM foods come from plants or animals that have been injected with DNA from a different species, causing them to produce new proteins that enable the food, say an apple, to grow quicker and stay firmer so it can be transported further. GM technology could, supposedly, be used to improve our food – pack our vegetables with more vitamins, for instance – but so far all it's done is benefit the producer.

Lazy girl's version: Food that has been changed on a chemical level. Genetic modification has not yet been fully tested, so we don't know what the impact will be on our health in 20 years.

Genito-Urinary Medicine (GUM) Clinics

Technical version: GUM clinics deal specifically with sexually transmitted infections such as HIV, chlamydia and genital bacterial infections. They are usually located in hospitals and are highly confidential. Records held at GUM clinics do not get sent to your GP or other clinics within the hospital.

Lazy girl's version: Sex or VD clinic.

Homeopathy

Technical version: Homeopathy is a method of helping the body heal itself. Homeopaths see the symptoms of an illness as the body's way of trying to overcome that particular condition. They therefore assist this process by using dilutions (made from plants) that mimic the illness. The quantities are so small that they heal rather than harm.

Lazy girl's version: Works well but in order to get the full benefits you have to give up coffee, tea and alcohol while taking the remedy. Ask yourself – is it worth it?

Good For:

- Skin conditions
- Headaches
- PMT
- Fatigue

Impotence

Technical version: Also known as erectile dysfunction, impotence affects 1 in 10 men on a regular basis and is

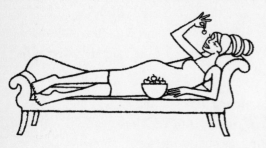

very common in men with high levels of anxiety and/or fatigue. The good news is that it's treatable and almost never serious.

Lazy girl's version: In men aged 20–40 impotence is usually the result of bad health, stress, tiredness or too much alcohol. Let him get some rest, make him improve his health and your sex life will improve.

Jet Lag

Technical version: The body's biological clock becomes desynchronised when you travel rapidly through different time zones. This leads to sleep problems, stomach problems, mental performance problems, fatigue and low energy. It takes a few days to acclimatise and then things get back to normal.

Lazy girl's versions: Beat jet lag by making sure you sleep at the right local hour even if you know it's really midnight at home. Experts also say that going out into bright sunlight as soon as you arrive in the new time zone helps your body get into the swing of things.

Kinesiology

Technical version: A procedure which involves testing muscles to identify weaknesses. Practitioners believe muscle groups are related to parts of the body and organs, so by identifying weak areas, illnesses and conditions can be diagnosed. Treatment is via dietary advice and supplements.

Lazy girl's version: Lots of lifting of legs and arms and pushing against the practitioner's 'resistance'. Might seem faintly hocus-pocus but devotees claim it can work a treat.

Good For:

- Food allergies
- Food intolerance

Liposuction

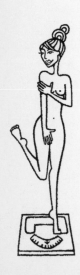

Technical version: A cosmetic surgery procedure whereby a tube is stuck into a small incision in the skin and fat tissue is literally vacuumed out. Generally used on inner thighs, bottoms, chins and stomachs. It's painful – and if you go in for 'debulking' (the removal of 15 kg (33lbs) or more in one go), potentially fatal.

Lazy girl's version: Think of a vacuum cleaner sucking fat out of your body . . .

Good For:

- Shaping specific areas of the body

Meditation

Technical version: A mental discipline whereby you learn to control your thoughts and calm the body to achieve a state of clarity and peace. Perfect for those who live with a high level of anxiety, insomnia and tension. It takes a few weeks to get the hang of, and can then be performed daily.

Lazy girl's version: Proven to help with relaxation and everything from PMT to panic attacks.

Good For:
- Highly-strung people
- Panic attacks
- Anxiety
- Insomnia

Metabolic rate

Technical version: The body's metabolic rate is the rate at which it burns calories for energy. Exercise regularly and eat healthily and you'll never feel the need to diet.

Lazy girl's version: Crash diet, starve yourself, yo-yo diet and you'll have to work harder to burn off normal amounts of energy and fat because your metabolic rate will dip and start working at a slower pace.

Naturopathy

Technical version: Naturopaths work by taking a holistic approach to illness: they look at the physical, psychological, nutritional and environmental factors in your whole life.

Lazy girl's version: For total wellbeing a naturopath may suggest you change your diet, take supplements and get some exercise.

Olestra

Technical version: Olestra is a fat substitute used in food. Supposedly the next big thing in diet control, the makers promise you can eat Olestra-coated fries and crisps and not get fat.

Lazy girl's version: Sadly, Olestra food has its drawbacks – in particular a reputation for what is delicately known as anal leakage.

Organic Food

Technical version: Food that has been grown naturally without the use of pesticides or GM technology.

Lazy girl's version: Food that looks grubby and oddly shaped in the shops but is natural and, therefore, better for your health (but not your purse).

Osteoporosis

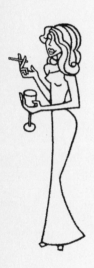

Technical version: Osteoporosis affects the trabecular bone – the spongy bone – between the hard outer crust and bone marrow, and is the part of the bone that naturally thins with age. No matter how fit and healthy you are, your bones will reach their maximum strength by your early 30s. After this, you'll start to lose bone mass at an approximate rate of 1% a year.

If you haven't developed a very high bone density by this time – due to lack of calcium, a poor diet, smoking, drinking, steroid treatment (for asthma) and basically being a couch potato – you may be at risk from developing osteoporosis.

Lazy girl's version: Want to avoid shrinking and broken bones? Then keep up an active lifestyle that includes some form of weight-bearing exercise (running, walking or weight training).

Pelvic Floor Exercises (Kegels)

Technical version: Do these exercises every day to strengthen your pubococcygeus (pelvic floor) muscles. You'll have a better sex life and avoid incontinence in later life.

Lazy girl's version: Clench and release the muscles you pee with (your pelvic floor muscles) 20 times a day.

Advocates swear you'll be in such good shape down below you'll be able to fire ping-pong balls.

Pelvic Inflammatory Disease

Technical version: An umbrella term for inflammation of the pelvic area caused by an infection, usually one that began in the cervix and has spread upwards. It can lead to problems with fertility and is often caused by the STI chlamydia.

Lazy girl's version: Discharge, pain during sex, fever and various other symptoms in the pelvic region. If this sounds familiar get checked out ASAP.

Pilates

Technical version: Endorsed by dancers and doctors for over a century, Pilates is a mind-body exercise regime that's akin to a very dynamic form of yoga. It's based on building a strong core group of muscles, body realignment and resistance work (against your own body weight).

Lazy girl's version: More like a supermodel exercise.

Refined Foods

Technical version: Foods that are no longer in their 'whole' state, and are pre-packaged, usually with added sugars, fats and white flours. They have little nutritional value and only add bad fats to your diet.

Lazy girl's version: Junk food – good for an instant pick me up, bad for your waistline and energy levels.

Reflexology

Technical version: The practice of applying pressure to points on the feet and hands (which correspond to areas of the body) to stimulate the body's own healing system.

Lazy girl's version: A deep foot massage with added health benefits.

Good For:

- Headaches
- Stress

Rosaeca

Technical version: Pronounced rose-ay-shah, this is a disease that affects the skin and leads to flushed patches on the face. It usually starts off looking like sunburn or acne but can spread along the cheeks, forehead and chin making the face look very red. See your GP for advice and medication.

Lazy girl's version: Control the redness by spotting your triggers: alcohol, chocolate, spicy foods, stress, sunlight and extreme temperatures can all make the condition worse. It also helps to choose make up and creams that won't clog your pores, such as non-comedogenic products.

Safe Period

Technical version: The stage in your menstrual cycle when you're least likely to get pregnant. Used by women who practise the rhythm method as a means of contraception.

Lazy girl's version: Not necessarily such a safe time to have sex if you can't be bothered to work out your cycle exactly, take your temperature daily and check mucus levels.

Stress

Technical version: The term used to describe added pressure in your life. It may come in the form of emotional problems, and/or work commitments, or be caused by upset plans, someone's behaviour, moving house, getting married or being ill – the list is endless.

Lazy girl's version: All those annoying commitments you have to face every day.

Toxic Shock Syndrome (TSS)

tips

Protect yourself from the risk of toxic shock syndrome by ensuring you use an absorbency that's right for your flow.

Technical version: A type of blood poisoning that is rare but potentially fatal. It's caused by a common bacterium that usually lives harmlessly on the body. Half of the reported cases (about 20 a year) happen in women using tampons with a high absorbency. It's recommended that women change their tampons frequently and, when using one over night, put a fresh one in before sleep and change it on waking.

Lazy girl's version: Extremely rare illness. The real scare was in the US over twenty years ago and was associated with a local brand of tampons. However, to protect yourself from the risk of TSS make sure you change your tampon regularly and choose an absorbency that's right for your flow.

UVA/UVB Rays

Technical version: The sun's ultraviolet rays. UVB are the rays that burn your skin and UVA rays are the ones that speed up the ageing process and cause skin cancer. In order to protect yourself you need a sunscreen that offers protection from both. Remember that UVA rays can damage your skin even on a cloudy day.

Lazy girl's version: Wear sunscreen with a sun protection factor (SPF) of no less that 15 in the summer, in hot climates and when it's sunny.

Vitamins

Technical version: These naturally occurring substances are essential for a healthy body and life. The best way to get them is through your food because this aids their absorption and helps them to work effectively. However, many foods do not contain the recommended daily allowance (RDA) as they lose some of their vitamin content either in preparation or cooking, so supplements are advised.

Lazy girl's version: All the nutrients you avoid if you only follow a low calorie, or junk and alcohol-based diet.

Warts (genital)

Technical version: Also known as HPV, genital warts are the fastest growing STI in the UK. They appear as small painless lumps around and in the genital area and need to be burnt off or treated by a doctor. Genital warts have been implicated in some cervical cancer cases so it's essential to have them treated as soon as possible.

Lazy girl's version: Cauliflower-like genital bumps.

Worms

Technical version: Enterobius vermicularis – or tiny white worms that inhabit the gut in one in three of us. They are caught by eating uncooked food or from other people, which is why you should always wash your hands after going to the toilet. See your pharmacist for anti-worm medication.

Lazy girl's version: Avoid BBQs and scrub under your nails with a nailbrush and you'll never be bothered by the wriggly blighters.

Xenical

Technical version: Xenical, also known as orlistat, is the new anti-obesity drug available on the NHS. It works by preventing fat from being absorbed in the body. However, it is vital to follow a low calorie, fat-free diet while taking it or you're asking for major stomach problems.

Lazy girl's version: Sadly not a miracle diet pill. You will only be prescribed it if you're classified obese, and too much pigging while taking it can lead to an instant evacuation of your bowels.

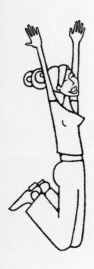

Yo-Yo Dieting

Technical version: Yo-yo dieting refers to the process of losing and gaining weight in repeated cycles. It can lead to an increased risk of heart disease, diabetes and more body fat than muscle.

Lazy girl's version: Being a diet bore.

Zzzz . . . Sleep

Technical version: Sleep is our natural state of rest and is essential if you want to be healthy, unstressed, physically fit and happy. Aim for 7–9 hours a night and you'll be fighting fit.

Lazy girl's version: Something you can do without getting off the couch AND it's actually good for you!

Where to go for help, advice and information

UK

Alcohol Concern, Waterbridge House, 32–36 Loman Street, London SE1 OEE
Tel: 020 7928 7377 Website: www.alcoholconcern.org.uk

Alcoholics Anonymous Tel: 020 7833 0022
Website: www.alcoholics-anonymous.org.uk

Alexander Technique (Society of AT Teachers), 20 London House, 266 Fulham
Road, London SW10 9EL Tel: 020 7351 0828 Website: www.stat.org.uk

ASH (Action on Smoking and Health), 102 Clifton Street, London EC2A 4HW
Tel: 020 7739 5902 Website: www.ash.org.uk

Association of Personal Trainers, PO Box 6131, London SW9 9XR
Tel: 020 8692 4023

Breast Cancer Care Helpline Tel: 0500 245345

British Association of Counselling, 1 Regents Place, Rugby CV21 2PJ
Tel: 01788 550899 Website: www.counselling.co.uk

British Dental Association (to find a dentist) Website: www.bda-dentistry.org.uk

British Heart Foundation, 14 Fitzhardinge Street, London W1H 6DH
Tel: 020 7935 0185 Website: www.bhf.org.uk

British Massage Therapy Council, 17 Rymers Lane, Oxford OX4 3JU
Tel: 01865 744123 Website: www.bmtc.co.uk

British Nutrition Foundation, High Holborn House, 52–54 High Holborn, London
WC1V 6RQ Tel: 020 7404 6504 Website: www.nutrition.org.uk

British Snoring and Sleep Apnoea Helpline (BSSAA) Send an SAE to: How Lane,
Chipstead, Surrey CR5 3LT Tel: 01737 557997

Centre for Stress Management, 156 Westcombe Hill, Blackheath, London SE23 7DH
Tel: 020 8293 4114 Website: www.managingstress.com

Depression Alliance Tel: 020 7633 0557 Website: www.depressionalliance.org

Diabetes Helpline Tel: 0207 636 6112 Website: www.diabetes.org.uk

Digestive Disorders Foundation Helpline Tel: 020 7487 5332

Drinkline Tel: 0345 320202

Eating Disorders Association, 1st Floor, Wensum House, 103 Prince of Wales Road,
Norwich, Norfolk NR1 1DW Tel: 01603 619090 Website: www.edauk.com

Family Planning Association, 2–12 Pentonville Road, London N1 9FP
Tel: 0845 310 1334 Website: www.fpa.org.uk

GUM Clinics NHS Direct Tel: 0845 4647 Website: www.nhsdirect.nhs.uk

Marie Stopes International (for sexual health and family planning clinics) Tel: 020 7388 0662

Migraine Action, Unit 6, Oakley Hay Lodge Business Park, Great Folds Road, Great Oakley, Northants NN18 9AS Tel: 01536 461333 Website: www.migraine.org.uk

Mind (National Association for Mental Health), 15–19 Broadway, London E15 4BQ Tel: 020 8522 1728 Website: www.mind.org.uk

National AIDS Helpline Tel: 0800 567123

National Association for Pre-menstrual Syndrome Helpline Tel: 01732 760 012

National Back Pain Association, 16 Elmtree Road, Teddington, Middx TW11 8FT Tel: 020 8977 5474 Website: www.backpain.org

National Centre for Eating Disorders, 54 New Road, Esher, Surrey KT10 9NO Tel: 01372 469493 Website: www.eating-disorders.org.uk

National Drugs Helpline Tel: 0800 776600

National Endometriosis Society Send an SAE to: 50 Westminster Palace Gardens, Artillery Row, London SW1P 1RL Tel: 020 7222 2776

National Osteoporosis Society, PO Box 10, Radstock, Bath BA3 3YB Tel: 01761 471104 Website: www.nos.org.uk

NHS Direct Tel: 0845 4647 Website: www.nhsdirect.nhs.uk

NO PANIC Helpline (for panic and anxiety attacks) Tel: 01952 590545

Quitline (smoking) Tel: 0800 002200

SAD (Seasonal Affective Disorder) Association, PO Box 969, London SW7 2PZ Tel: 01903 814942 Website: www.sada.org.uk

Samaritans National Helpline Tel: 08457 909090

Women's Nutritional Advisory Service, PO Box 268, Lewes, East Sussex BN7 1QN
Tel: 01273 487366 Website: www.wnas.org.uk

Australia

Australian Natural Therapists Association Tel: 1800 817 577
Website: www.anta.com.au

Eating Disorders Association Helpline: (02) 9899 5344
Website: www.edansw.org.au

Family Planning Queensland, 9/114 Maitland Street, Hackett, ACT 2602
Tel: (02) 6230 5255 Website: www.fpq.asn.au

Mental Health Association of Australia Website: www.mentalhealth.org.au

New Zealand

Auckland Sexual Health Service (ASHS), Building 16, Auckland Hospital,
Park Road, Grafton Tel: (09) 307 2885 Website: www.sexfiles.co.nz

Community Alcohol and Drug Service (CADS) Tel: (09) 815 5830
Website: www.whl.co.nz/sorted

South Africa

Cancer Association of South Africa, PO Box 186, Rondebosch 7701
Tel: (021) 689 5381 Tol free: 0800 226 622 Website: www.cansa.org.za

Medical Research Council of South Africa, PO Box 19070, 7505 Tygerberg
Website: www.mrc.ac.za

index